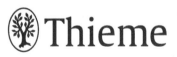

Emerging Technologies in Face and Body Contouring

Spero J. Theodorou, MD
Clinical Assistant Professor of Surgery
Donald and Barbara Zucker School of Medicine
Hofstra/Northwell, Hempstead, New York;
Teaching Faculty
Aesthetic Plastic Surgery Fellowship
Manhattan Eye, Ear, and Throat Hospital;
Surgical Director and Co-Founder
bodySCULPT Plastic Surgery
New York, New York, USA

Christopher T. Chia, MD
Clinical Assistant Professor of Surgery
Donald and Barbara Zucker School of Medicine
Hofstra/Northwell, Hempstead, New York;
Teaching Faculty
Aesthetic Plastic Surgery Fellowship
Manhattan Eye, Ear, and Throat Hospital;
Surgical Director and Co-Founder
bodySCULPT Plastic Surgery
New York, New York, USA

Erez Dayan, MD
Harvard Trained Plastic Surgeon
Medical Director of Avance Plastic Surgery Institute
Reno/Tahoe, Nevada and Los Angeles, California, USA

353 illustrations

Thieme
New York • Stuttgart • Delhi • Rio de Janeiro

Library of Congress Cataloging-in-Publication Data is available from the publisher

Important note: Medicine is an ever-changing science undergoing continual development. Research and clinical experience are continually expanding our knowledge, in particular our knowledge of proper treatment and drug therapy. Insofar as this book mentions any dosage or application, readers may rest assured that the authors, editors, and publishers have made every effort to ensure that such references are in accordance with **the state of knowledge at the time of production of the book.**

Nevertheless, this does not involve, imply, or express any guarantee or responsibility on the part of the publishers in respect to any dosage instructions and forms of applications stated in the book. **Every user is requested to examine carefully** the manufacturers' leaflets accompanying each drug and to check, if necessary, in consultation with a physician or specialist,whether the dosage schedules mentioned therein or the contraindications stated by the manufacturers differ from the statements made in the present book. Such examination is particularly important with drugs that are either rarely used or have been newly released on the market. Every dosage schedule or every form of application used is entirely at the user's own risk and responsibility. The authors and publishers request every user to report to the publishers any discrepancies or inaccuracies noticed. If errors in this work are found after publication, errata will be posted at www.thieme.com on the product description page.

Some of the product names, patents, and registered designs referred to in this book are in fact registered trademarks or proprietary names even though specific reference to this fact is not always made in the text. Therefore, the appearance of a name without designation as proprietary is not to be construed as a representation by the publisher that it is in the public domain.

© 2021. Thieme. All rights reserved.

Thieme Medical Publishers, Inc.
333 Seventh Avenue, 18th Floor
New York, NY 10001, USA
www.thieme.com
+1 800 782 3488, customerservice@thieme.com

Cover design: Thieme Publishing Group
Typesetting by DiTech Process Solutions, India

Printed in USA by King Printing Company, Inc.   5 4 3 2 1

ISBN 978-1-62-623667-7

Also available as an e-book:
eISBN 978-1-62-623879-4

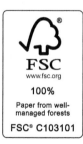

FSC
www.fsc.org
100%
Paper from well-managed forests
FSC® C103101

To John Polley for his belief in me, Nick Tabbal for his generous friendship, and Daniel Baker for his valuable guidance and support. To Gerald Pitman, for introducing me to the art of liposuction and to all the teachers who contributed to my education as a plastic surgeon. To my father, John, for allowing me to dream unencumbered. To my mother, Maria, for her stalwart belief in me while always stressing on the realities of my predicament, and my brother, Peter, for the endless love and scars on my head to go with it. To my amazing wife, Julie, for hanging in there through the insanity and sticking with me despite her best judgement to flee for the hills. Lastly, to my daughter, Mary, for bringing me to my knees and my son, John, for delivering the final blow to any remaining vestiges of ego that I held on to. I love you all to the moon and back. "Pan Metron Ariston" aside.

Spero J. Theodorou

To my wife, Melissa, for her unwavering support throughout the years with whom I took this journey with so many unexpected twists and turns. To my children, Annalise and Nico, through whose eyes I see the fresh perspective of limitless opportunities, and to my mother Sophie and father Frank, who instilled in me the strength to overcome even the most daunting challenges. I also wish to thank my plastic surgery teachers who provided me with the tools and skills to humbly carry on the privilege of our specialty to the best of my ability.

Christopher T. Chia

To my parents, Shalom and Simcha Dayan, who immigrated to this country with nothing, and gave my brother and me everything. Thank you for believing in us before we believed in ourselves. To my brother, Etan, for sharing this journey with me. To my wife, Tali, for being my life's co-pilot and family's foundation. I could not have dreamed of a better mother and life partner; without you this wouldn't be possible. To my sons, Elon, Asher, and Leor—you make each day more exciting than the next. Your love and energy helped me get my second wind. To John and Catherine Farahi, thank you for your unconditional love and support; I could not have asked for better second parents. Lastly, to my co-authors, Dr. Spero J. Theodorou and Dr. Christopher Chia for their support throughout my career as a plastic surgeon.

Erez Dayan

Contents

Contents

Section IV   Technology-Based Body Contouring by Anatomy

Contents

Contents

Foreword

When introduced approximately 40 years ago, liposuction was a revolutionary concept. Though highly effective in reducing regional body fat, its results were relatively crude and lacked the control associated with traditional surgery.

Subsequent refinements, using thinner cannulas and safer local anesthetic techniques have made it the most popular procedure in aesthetic plastic surgery.

In spite of its success and popularity, liposuction has always had significant limitations, primarily in relation to the lack of control of the skin envelope. The skilled operator would be constantly assessing the new relationship between the subcutaneous dead space created by the procedure and the ability of the overlying skin to adapt to the new contour. The patient's age, area being treated, and a multitude of other factors play a role in determining the ability of the skin envelope to retract properly. These parameters often played a limiting role in terms of achieving ideal outcomes.

Today's patients have high expectations. They seek nonsurgical treatments when available and tend to avoid procedures associated with prolonged recovery time. Over the past few years, new technologies have emerged—using lasers, ultrasound technology, radiofrequency waves, and a new variety of means to dissolve fat cells without surgery. These modalities have radically expanded the field of body contouring by enhancing the ability of the skin to retract, while reducing surgical morbidity. This pioneering book, edited by Dr. Theodorou, Dr. Chia, and Dr. Dayan introduces this new chapter in the science of body contouring. I am thrilled to see Dr. Theodorou and Dr. Chia take the lead in this new field. Having had a hand in their surgical education, I look at their accomplishments with excitement and genuine pride.

Nicolas Tabbal, MD
Clinical Associate Professor of Surgery
Institute of Reconstructive Plastic Surgery
New York University School of Medicine
New York, New York, USA

Preface

Technological advances over the past decade have transformed the aesthetic landscape. From patient analysis to treatment and postoperative care—the manner in which aesthetic treatment is provided today is vastly different than it was in the times of our predecessors. In addition, aesthetic providers are increasingly coming from more diverse training backgrounds, often with a paucity of training in aesthetic technology.

In this book, the latest aesthetic techniques have been discussed with theoretical and practical guidelines. It will serve as a curated guide for the clinicians. The contributors of this book are recognized clinical experts. They have provided concise yet comprehensive details in their areas of expertise for optimal use and safety.

We hope that the readers will find this unique work as a valuable resource to deepen their understanding of emerging aesthetic technology and broaden their practice armamentarium.

Spero J. Theodorou, MD
Christopher T. Chia, MD
Erez Dayan, MD

Contributors

Sherrell J. Aston, MD, FACS
Chairman
Department of Plastic Surgery
Manhattan Eye Ear and Throat Hospital;
Professor
Department of Plastic Surgery
New York University
New York City, New York, USA

William G. Austen Jr., MD, FACS
Chief
Division of Plastic and Reconstructive Surgery and Division of
    Burn Surgery
Massachusetts General Hospital
Boston, Massachusetts, USA

Anne Chapas, MD
Director
Union Square Laser Dermatology
Instructor of Dermatology
Mount Sinai Medical Center
New York, New York, USA

Christopher T. Chia, MD
Clinical Assistant Professor of Surgery
Donald and Barbara Zucker School of Medicine
Hofstra/Northwell, Hempstead, New York;
Teaching Faculty
Aesthetic Plastic Surgery Fellowship
Manhattan Eye, Ear, and Throat Hospital;
Surgical Director and Co-Founder
bodySCULPT Plastic Surgery
New York, New York, USA

Jennifer Croix, MD, PhD
Board Certified Dermatologist
Illinois Dermatology Institute
Skokie, Illinois, USA

Erez Dayan, MD
Harvard Trained Plastic Surgeon
Medical Director of Avance Plastic Surgery Institute
Reno/Tahoe, Nevada and Los Angeles, California, USA

John W. Decorato, MD, FACS
Board Certified Plastic Surgeon
Medical Director
Aesthetic Pavilion Ambulatory Surgery Center
Richmond, New York, USA

Briar L. Dent, MD
Plastic and Reconstructive Surgeon
Westmed Medical Group
Purchase, New York, USA

Diane Irvine Duncan, MD, FACS
Plastic Surgeon
Plastic Surgical Associates of Fort Collins
Fort Collins, Colorado, USA

Rachel L. Goldstein, DO
Plastic Surgery Fellow, PGY-6
Houston Methodist Hospital
Houston, Texas, USA

David E. Guarin, MD
Plastic Surgeon
Professor
Plastic Surgery Section
PLASTICUV Research Group
Universidad del Valle
Cali, Colombia

Alfredo Hoyos, MD
Associate Professor
Department of Plastic Surgery
University of San Martin in Bogota
Bogotá, Colombia

Evangelos Keramidas, MD, FEBOPRAS
Director
Department of Plastic, Aesthetic, and Reconstructive Surgery
Co-Founder of Kosmesis Aesthetic Plastic Surgery Center
Central Clinic of Athens
Athens, Greece

William Lao, MD
Board Certified Plastic Surgeon
Private Practice
New York, New York, USA

Steven M. Levine, MD
Clinical Assistant Professor of Plastic Surgery
Zucker School of Medicine at Hofstra University
New York, New York, USA

Sophie Pei-Hsuan Lu, MD
Director
Haute Age Aesthetic Medicine Clinic
Former Assistant Professor
Department of Dermatology and Aesthetic Medical Center
Chang Gung Memorial Hospital
Taipei, Taiwan

W. Jason Martin, MD
Board Certified Plastic Surgeon
Adjunct Professor
Department of Plastic Surgery
University of Colorado
Denver, Colorado, USA

Alix O'Brien, PA-C
NCCPA Board Certified Physician
New York, New York, USA

Mauricio Perez, MD
Plastic Surgeon
Private Practice
Bogotá, Colombia

Gerald H. Pitman, MD
Cosmetic, Plastic, and Reconstructive Surgery Specialist
President
Gerald H Pitman MD PC
New York, New York, USA

B. Aviva Preminger, MD, MPH, FACS
Preminger Plastic Surgery
Department of Surgery
Columbia University
New York City, New York, USA

Contributors

Isabel Robinson, MD
Resident
The Hansjörg Wyss Department of Plastic Surgery
NYU Grossman School of Medicine
New York, New York, USA

Villy Rodopoulou, MD, FEBOPRAS
Consultant Plastic Surgeon
Co-Founder of Kosmesis Aesthetic Plastic Surgery Center
Department of Plastic, Aesthetic, and Reconstructive Surgery
Central Clinic of Athens
Athens, Greece

P. Paolo Rovatti, MD
Lecturer
Agorà (School of Aesthetic Medicine)
International College of Aesthetic Medicine (ICAMP)
Founder and Director
Studio Rovatti Clinic
Verona, Italy

Pierre Saadeh, MD
Vice Chair for Education
Associate Professor
The Hansjörg Wyss Department of Plastic Surgery
NYU Grossman School of Medicine
Chief of Plastic Surgery
Department of Plastic Surgery
Bellevue Hospital
New York, New York, USA

Douglas Senderoff, MD, FACS
Board Certified Plastic Surgeon
Park Avenue Aesthetic Surgery
New York, New York, USA

Sachin M. Shridharani, MD, FACS
Board Certified Plastic Surgeon
Founder of LUXURGERY–The Confluence of Luxury and
  Aesthetic Surgery
New York City, New York, USA

Aris Sterodimas, MD, MSc, PhD, ARCS
Head
Department of Plastic and Reconstructive Surgery
Metropolitan General Hospital in Athens
Athens, Greece

Spero J. Theodorou, MD
Clinical Assistant Professor of Surgery
Donald and Barbara Zucker School of Medicine
Hofstra/Northwell, Hempstead, New York;
Teaching Faculty
Aesthetic Plastic Surgery Fellowship
Manhattan Eye, Ear, and Throat Hospital;
Surgical Director and Co-Founder
bodySCULPT Plastic Surgery
New York, New York, USA

Steven Hsiang-Ya Wang, MD
Director
Taipei Arts Plastic Clinic
Taipei, Taiwan

Stelios C. Wilson, MD
Aesthetic Surgery Fellow
Department of Plastic Surgery
Manhattan Eye, Ear, and Throat Hospital
New York, New York, USA

Section I

Principles

I

1 Three-dimensional Imaging for Emerging Technologies in Body Contouring

Isabel Robinson and Pierre Saadeh

Abstract

Initially adopted by craniofacial surgeons, three-dimensional imaging technology has more recently expanded into the fields of breast and body contouring. These systems create value pre-, intra-, and postoperatively by facilitating a more objective conversation with patients on preoperative expectations, enabling the creation of personalized cutting guides and implants, and allowing surgeons to more accurately quantify their results over time. While currently limited by cost and technical training requirements, as these technologies continue to develop they are likely to become an indispensable resource in the body contouring surgeon's armamentarium.

Keywords: Three-dimensional (3D) imaging, CADCAS, body contouring, cephalometrics, mammometrics, ultrahigh-sensitive optical microangiography

Key Points

- Summary of 3D imaging technologies' technical points, applications, and points for consideration (▶ Table 1.1).

Table 1.1 Summary of 3D imaging technologies' technical points, applications, and points for consideration

Patient selection	Indications/contraindications: all standard body contouring indications/contraindications apply, specifics vary by procedure(s)
Technique	The patient is photographed (still or in motion depending on the desired information), and a digital image is created. Depending on the system, anatomical landmarks are automatically or manually identified. Landmarks can then be manipulated to alter the image, giving an idea of potential surgical outcomes. Postoperative images can be taken and compared to preoperative images to give quantitative data on volumetric changes
Clinical applications	Preoperatively, imaging can be used to consult the patient on the aesthetic outcomes of potential procedures. Intraoperatively, it can be used to create 3D-printed models, implants, and cutting guides. Postoperatively, it can be used to quantitatively assess outcomes and to monitor changes over time
Combinations with other technologies	Imaging complements all soft tissue manipulations, particularly for face and breast as relatively extensive literature exists in these two areas. Principles can be applied to other body areas but will likely require greater manual effort on the part of the user as fewer automated analysis systems exist for these areas
Pros	• Quantitative, objective assessment • Automatic landmark identification and volume analysis more efficient than manual calculation • Increased patient trust and satisfaction
Cons	• Cost ($20,000–$60,000) • Technological training required • Current software mainly focused on face/breast

1.1 Introduction

3D imaging is a powerful emerging technology in the field of body contouring. Body contouring inherently deals with three-dimensional changes and relationships, and yet preoperative planning and postoperative assessment has historically relied on two-dimensional representations. With the advent of 3D imaging, volumetric analysis can be performed and visualized with an accuracy that 2D photographs are incapable of meeting. This enables surgeons to give patients a better understanding of their likely surgical outcomes and to ensure mutual understanding about surgical goals. It also provides a quantitative means of assessing outcomes and volume-based changes over time in order to further refine technique and optimize surgical outcomes. Newly-developing 3D imaging technologies are advancing the understanding of microvasculature[1] and allowing surgeons and patients to experiment with various aesthetic outcomes using virtual simulations in real time.[2] 3D imaging revolutionizes the way surgeons are able to visualize patient data and holds great potential for both clinical and research applications.

1.2 History of 3D Imaging in Plastic Surgery

The history of 3D imaging begins with stereophotogrammetry, the practice of estimating three-dimensional coordinates on an object's surface by using photographs of the object taken from different positions. The technique affords a more nuanced understanding of three-dimensional and volumetric relationships than traditional two-dimensional photography. Mannsbach originally suggested applying stereophotogrammetry to the fields of medicine and dentistry in 1922, and in 1939 Zeller first published a contour map of a man's face using a stereocamera.[3] It was not until 1944, however, that stereophotogrammetry was applied in a clinical setting, with Thalmann using the technique to diagnose orthodontic pathology.[3]

Since then many variations upon the technique have developed, most notably computer-assisted systems that greatly improve the speed and depth of analysis. Such advances include optical flow tracking, which incorporates time into three-dimensional analyses to give the user the ability to track soft tissue changes immediately during motion or longitudinally after surgery. One such iteration is 3D speckle tracking, in which white makeup is first applied to the patient's face or other surfaces of interest. Black makeup is then dotted over the white, creating a speckled appearance that a computer can detect. In a craniofacial case, the patient then makes a series of facial expressions that displace the speckles while the computer tracks and analyzes these changes, producing a report on the patient's facial expressivity. Newer technologies, such as the Di4D optical flow tracking software (Glasgow, Scotland), are able to track facial motion by digitally creating a mesh over a patient's face and tracing changes to it over time, thereby obviating the need for makeup application. One of the newest developments in the field of three-dimensional medical imaging is ultrahigh sensitive optical microangiography (UHS-OMAG), with which Doppler monitoring of blood cell movement is able to produce 3D maps of capillary microvasculature in the skin after five seconds of scanning.[1]

What follows will be a review of current clinical applications of three-dimensional imaging technologies like optical flow tracking and UHS-OMAG to the practice of body contouring. Applications to breast and facial surgery will be emphasized as the majority of existent research on 3D imaging technologies comes from these subspecialties. However, many of the principles discussed apply equally to most body contouring procedures.

1.3 Preoperative Benefit of 3D Imaging

As early as 1978, computer-assisted cephalometric readings were described by Malmgren et al, as a means of quantifying the appearance of bony structures in the head.[4] In 1987, Guyuron expanded the concept of cephalometrics into soft-tissue analysis, describing quantitative standards for measuring the nose to aid in rhinoplasty planning.[5] Classical cephalometrics involves taking manual readings of anatomical landmarks and then tracing them by hand onto acetate paper to assess facial and dental harmony. Cephalometric planning has been used in the diagnosis and treatment planning of a wide range of craniofacial pathologies. The advent of digital cephalometric technology has dramatically increased the speed with which these measurements can be performed and the level of volumetric detail that can be assessed.[6] With a computer-assisted digital cephalometric analysis system (CADCAS), the patient's 3D image is captured through stereophotogrammetry. Software then automatically identifies facial landmarks and calculates relevant volumes and distances. Computer-assisted cephalometric measurements have been shown repeatedly to produce results that correlate strongly with manually-derived values.[6,7]

A challenge in aesthetic breast surgery is the lack of normative databases relative to craniofacial practice. Traditionally aesthetic breast surgery planning and outcome assessment has been based off qualitative discussion between the surgeon and patient. This makes developing digital assistance programs, which are inherent quantitative, difficult. Nevertheless, efforts have been made to standardize breast surgery evaluation with the aid of three-dimensional imaging. To this end, Karp et al describe the emerging principle of mammometrics as a tool for breast surgery planning and evaluation through three-dimensional volumetric analysis.[2] As with cephalometrics, mammometrics involves using 3D imaging systems to photograph the patient and then identifying key landmarks on the resulting three-dimensional representation. Unlike in craniofacial surgery, which has CADCAS systems that can automatically identify important landmarks, the development of 3D breast imaging systems is relatively new and so automatic image interpretation is still in its infancy. As such, for 3D breast imaging programs the surgeon must either fine-tune breast landmarks identified by the software or manually identify key landmarks from which the software derives relevant volumes. Karp et al suggest including total breast volume, volumetric distribution, and breast projection among the volume measures obtained.[2] Further studies have validated 3D imaging of the breast to show accuracy of volume measurements by the software on mastectomy specimens within 2% of measured volume, accuracy of change in breast volume before and after augmentation, as well as accuracy of automated measurements of up to 91%.[8,9,10,11]

Once the images are captured and landmarks labeled, both craniofacial and breast 3D images provide significant benefit to the surgeon for preoperative planning. Digitally-obtained and labeled images have the advantage of being more easily manipulated, and 3D images provide important information on volumes and spatial relationships that standard 2D photographs are unable to match. This gives the surgeon realistic visual estimates of the aesthetic results that would be obtained by changing different volumetric values during surgery. Not only does this help the surgeon in preoperative planning, but it is a highly valuable tool during the patient consult for education and conversion to surgery. With the aid of 3D imaging, the surgeon can demonstrate the different aesthetic outcomes possible to give the patient a more precise and personalized understanding of what options are available to them. During a rhinoplasty consult, a surgeon can use a CADCAS to virtually manipulate the nasolabial angle, nasofrontal angle, nasal tip, and dorsal hump of the patient to demonstrate the effect of each procedure.[12] Similarly, software can demonstrate the 3D effects of breast augmentation surgery depending on the implant size and shape. Such planning helps check patient understanding, manage patient expectations, and allows a more quantitative set of goals for the surgery.

1.4 Intraoperative Benefit of 3D Imaging

In addition to the patient consult, three-dimensional imaging can help the surgeon intraoperatively by aiding in the creation of cutting guides and implants personally selected for the patient. In craniofacial surgery, lateral radiographs and CT scans can be converted into digital 3D images or 3D printed models of a patient's skull. Simulated surgeries can then be performed using these 3D images and models, giving the surgeon a more precise understanding of the specifics of the patient's anatomy and the degree to which tissues must be manipulated to achieve the desired outcome. Personalized cutting guides and fixation templates can be designed based on these simulated surgeries and then 3D printed according to each patient's unique measurements. When applied to genioplasty this system resulted in postoperative results that closely matched preoperative plans and very high overall patient satisfaction.[13] Three-dimensional imaging provides similar intraoperative benefits to breast surgery. For breast reduction, preoperative mammometric analysis can give the surgeon a quantitative goal for resection weight per breast, which can help ensure balance particularly in cases of significant preoperative asymmetry between the breasts.

Along with 3D virtual representations of surface anatomy, imaging systems now exist that are able to map in three dimensions underlying capillary beds, a powerful tool in soft tissue surgery. Ultrahigh sensitive optical microangiography offers substantial pre- and intraoperative benefits through its ability to quickly and precisely map facial microvasculature, producing three-dimensional images of capillary beds to facilitate research into vascular changes and wound healing. In one application, UHS-OMAG was used to demonstrate that morbidity from hyaluronic acid-based facial rejuvenation procedures can be caused by inadvertent injection of the filler into capillaries in the face.[14] The ability of this technology to produce accurate 3D representations of microanatomy enables the modeling of a wide range of surgical situations, and will continue to provide important information for reducing morbidity and improving surgical technique.

1.5 Postoperative Benefit of 3D Imaging

In addition to pre- and intraoperative benefits, 3D imaging technology holds immense value as a tool for quantitative postoperative assessment. This is especially true in the case of craniofacial surgery, for which extensive collections of normative data exist. 3D imaging allows surgeons to more readily quantify post-surgical cephalometric change and compare end results with the preoperative plan as well as normative data. 3D speckle tracking spectrophotogrammetry has been applied in this way to objectively measure the effects of botulinum toxin type A treatment for rhytids, with digitally-generated heatmaps demonstrating the change in motility across the face from pre- to postoperative.[15] Similarly, 3D image analysis was used to create the first-ever objective, quantitative demonstration of the long-term effectiveness of hyaluronic acid in tear trough rejuvenation.[16]

While there is not a comparable normative mammometric database to compare results to, three-dimensional imaging does give breast surgeons the ability to quantitatively assess the volumetric change achieved during surgery. Such assessment is critical for continuing to develop an evidence-based literature with which to judge the efficacy of surgical techniques and materials. Using pre- and postoperative 3D imaging, Karp et al demonstrated that the projection of 28 breasts following implant placement was 20.9% less than the manufacturer-reported projection.[17] In addition to quantifying immediately post-surgical results, three-dimensional imaging enables long-term assessment of surgical outcomes. In one study of reduction mammaplasty patients, 3D imaging demonstrated the process of pseudoptosis development in the first postoperative year as well as the resolution of the pseudoptosis in the second postoperative year.[18] In this way 3D imaging is able to record quantitatively long-term postoperative volumetric changes. Knowledge of these changes may aid in future surgical consultation and planning by giving physicians a more defined estimate of changes that are likely to occur after surgery.

1.6 Limitations

While novel 3D imaging technologies hold great potential for enhancing surgical planning and outcome assessment, they are not meant as a replacement for the trained surgical eye. Aesthetic procedures have an inherent level of subjectivity, and the quantitative contributions of 3D imaging and analysis systems supplement but do not substitute the qualitative judgment of the surgeon. Additionally, three-dimensional imaging systems may be prohibitively expensive, with 3D cameras typically costing between $20,000 and $60,000.[2] Lower cost alternatives include handheld, iPad-based models that can range from $1,000 to $10,000.[12] Analysis systems that depend on manual landmark identification, including all extant breast imaging systems, require the operator to be trained in using the software. The perceived user friendliness depends on the system chosen and the familiarity of the operator with digital image manipulation.

1.7 Conclusion

3D imaging is a powerful new tool with both research and clinical applications. Its value will continue to be demonstrated in pre-, intra-, and postoperative settings as its use becomes increasingly common. With three-dimensional imaging and analysis, body contouring practices can enhance the patient experience and contribute to the advancement of the field.

References

[1] An L, Qin J, Wang RK. Ultrahigh sensitive optical microangiography for in vivo imaging of microcirculations within human skin tissue beds. Opt Express 2010;18(8):8220–8228

[2] Tepper OM, Unger JG, Small KH, et al. Mammometrics: the standardization of aesthetic and reconstructive breast surgery. Plast Reconstr Surg 2010;125(1):393–400

[3] Burke PH, Beard FH. Stereophotogrammetry of the face. A preliminary investigation into the accuracy of a simplified system evolved for contour mapping by photography. Am J Orthod 1967;53(10):769–782

[4] Bergin R, Hallenberg J, Malmgren O. Computerized cephalometrics. Acta Odontol Scand 1978;36(6):349–357

[5] Guyuron B. Precision rhinoplasty. Part I: The role of life-size photographs and soft-tissue cephalometric analysis. Plast Reconstr Surg 1988;81(4):489–499

[6] Chen SK, Chen YJ, Yao CCJ, Chang HF. Enhanced speed and precision of measurement in a computer-assisted digital cephalometric analysis system. Angle Orthod 2004;74(4):501–507

[7] Heike CL, Cunningham ML, Hing AV, Stuhaug E, Starr JR. Picture perfect? Reliability of craniofacial anthropometry using three-dimensional digital stereophotogrammetry. Plast Reconstr Surg 2009;124(4):1261–1272

[8] Losken A, Seify H, Denson DD, Paredes AA Jr, Carlson GW. Validating three-dimensional imaging of the breast. Ann Plast Surg 2005;54(5):471–476, discussion 477–478

[9] Mailey B, Freel A, Wong R, Pointer DT, Khoobehi K. Clinical accuracy and reproducibility of Portrait 3D Surgical Simulation Platform in breast augmentation. Aesthet Surg J 2013;33(1):84–92

[10] Creasman CN, Mordaunt D, Liolios T, Chiu C, Gabriel A, Maxwell GP. Four-dimensional breast imaging, part I: introduction of a technology-driven, evidence-based approach to breast augmentation planning. Aesthet Surg J 2011;31(8):914–924

[11] Roostaeian J, Adams WP Jr. Three-dimensional imaging for breast augmentation: is this technology providing accurate simulations? Aesthet Surg J 2014;34(6):857–875

[12] Weissler JM, Stern CS, Schreiber JE, Amirlak B, Tepper OM. The evolution of photography and three-dimensional imaging in plastic surgery. Plast Reconstr Surg 2017;139(3):761–769

[13] Qiao J, Fu X, Gui L, et al. Computer image-guided template for horizontal advancement genioplasty. J Craniofac Surg 2016;27(8):2004–2008

[14] Chang SH, Yousefi S, Qin J, et al. External compression versus intravascular injection: a mechanistic animal model of filler-induced ischemia. Ophthal Plast Reconstr Surg 2016;32(4):261–266

[15] Wilson AJ, Chin BC, Hsu VM, Mirzabeigi MN, Percec I. Digital image correlation: a novel dynamic three-dimensional imaging technique for precise quantification of the dynamic rhytid and botulinum toxin type a efficacy. Plast Reconstr Surg 2015;135(5):869e–876e

[16] Donath AS, Glasgold RA, Meier J, Glasgold MJ. Quantitative evaluation of volume augmentation in the tear trough with a hyaluronic acid-based filler: a three-dimensional analysis. Plast Reconstr Surg 2010;125(5):1515–1522

[17] Tepper OM, Small KH, Unger JG, et al. 3D analysis of breast augmentation defines operative changes and their relationship to implant dimensions. Ann Plast Surg 2009;62(5):570–575

[18] Choi M, Unger J, Small K, et al. Defining the kinetics of breast pseudoptosis after reduction mammaplasty. Ann Plast Surg 2009;62(5):518–522

2 Clinically Applicable Concepts of Fat Metabolism

Rachel L. Goldstein, William G. Austen Jr., and Erez Dayan

Abstract

This chapter explores surgically applicable anatomical, compositional, and diverse physiologic properties of adipose tissue and their effects on outcomes after body contouring procedures. Adipose is a complex, active endocrine organ. Eighty five percent of all adipose tissue in the human body is subcutaneous, arranged into apical, mantle, and deep layers. The deep layer is found deep to Scarpa's fascia and is the target layer for liposuction. Adipose tissue is highly vascularized with low oxygen demand and high susceptibility to epinephrine in tumescent fluid. It contains a variety of cell types including a rich store of mesenchymal stem cells, adipocytes arranged into lobules, and supportive connective tissue. Now considered the largest endocrine organ in the body, adipose plays active roles in energy homeostasis, glucose metabolism, immune function, and hormonal regulation. According to the widely accepted "Lipostatic Hypothesis," the total body number of adipocytes is set during adolescence. Centrally regulated autonomic processes work to maintain a set body weight. If these are overwhelmed by a chronic positive or negative energy balance, adipocytes will change size and eventually volume with resultant metabolic sequelae. Some studies suggest that after lipectomy procedures, the lipostatic mechanism can lead to compensatory fat growth in non-surgically resected areas, both subcutaneous and visceral, beginning 3 months postoperatively. Potential resulting metabolic changes may theoretically affect the patient's overall health as a result. Finally, understanding the structure and biologic properties of the adipocyte will help guide surgical techniques to improve overall "take" after fat grafting procedures.

Keywords: Adipose tissue anatomy, lipectomy, obesity, fat homeostasis, fat biology, adipocyte, fat grafting

2.1 Introduction

While historically we thought that adipose was an inert tissue, capable only of energy storage, this over-simplified understanding is now a thing of the past. After extensive research in recent years, adipose is now regarded as a highly specialized, complex endocrine organ exerting widespread effects in virtually all organ systems. According to the American Society for Aesthetic Plastic Surgery, suction lipectomy has become the most common plastic surgery intervention, with almost 400,000 patients treated in 2015. Increases in this patient population further obligates surgeons of the adipose organ to master an understanding of its biology, which will in turn cultivate a deeper appreciation for liposculptural impact and afford improved results.[1]

2.2 Anatomy of Adipose Tissue

2.2.1 Gross Structure

Adipose tissue exists throughout the human body providing the largest volumetric contribution to the connective tissue matrix. Total body fat in lean adults, of which 85% is subcutaneous and the remaining is visceral, contributes approximately 8–18% of total body weight in males and 14–28% in females, and can reach up to 60–70% in obese patients.[2]

Markman and Barton were the first to investigate the gross anatomy of subcutaneous fat in a cadaveric study in 1987. Their findings are still commonly accepted and utilized today.[3] There are three discrete layers of subcutaneous fat: apical (or Periadnexal), mantle (or superficial), and deep.

The apical layer is most superficial, located just beneath the reticular dermis, containing yellow-appearing fat and fibrous septa running perpendicular to the skin. Other structures are present including sweat glands, hair follicles, and vascular and lymphatic channels. All these structures are susceptible to damage by the liposuction cannula if this layer is not carefully avoided (▶ Fig. 2.1). Traumatic injuries were more common when larger diameter cannulas were used (8–10 mm) with sequelae including seromas, hyperpigmentation, and even skin necrosis. These complications are rare in today's era of 2–3 mm cannulas.[3,4]

Next is the mantle layer, located everywhere but the eyelids, nail beds, bridge of the nose, and penis, and containing small fat lobules packed tightly with closely-spaced septae. It serves as a shock absorber, helping the skin resist trauma by distributing pressure over a larger field. The thickness of this layer is consistent throughout the body and correlates with the "pinch test", a depth gauge for the liposuction cannula which should be inserted just beneath this layer.[3,4,5]

Finally, the deep layer, situated just above the underlying muscle fascia, contains large, irregular, poorly organized fat lobules. It is separated from the mantle layer by a continuous fibroelastic membrane, the fascia superficialis (called Scarpa's, Colles', or Camper's fascia in certain anatomic areas). This is

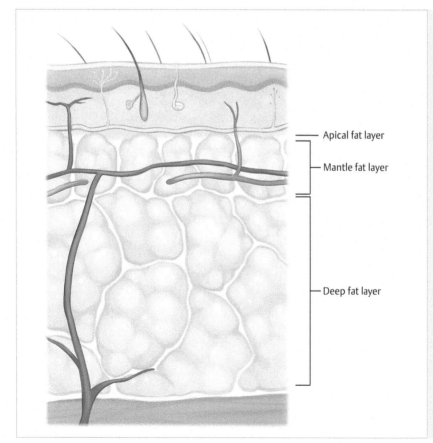

Apical fat layer

Mantle fat layer

Deep fat layer

Fig. 2.1 Lipocyte distribution from the dermis to the muscular fascia. Damage to the apical and mantle layers represent may compromise the blood supply to the skin and predispose to postoperative complications such as seroma or dermal necrosis.

target layer for liposuction. Its thickness varies by region based on genetics, diet, and sex, with distinct gender-specific distributions to consider during body contouring procedures. While females display a metabolically-favorable gynoid or peripheral distribution, with increased fat deposition in the glute-ofemoral areas, men tend toward a metabolically-unfavorable android or central distribution with increased visceral deposition.[6]

2.2.2 Cellular Components and Structure

A wide variety of cell types comprise the adipose organ, of which only an estimated 50% are actually adipocytes (▶Fig. 2.2).[2] Other cells that intermingle with the predominant adipocyte, including preadipocytes, endothelial cells, smooth muscle cells, and fibroblasts, are essential to the structure and function of adipose. Stem cells also exist in quantities so rich that adipose is considered their largest known reservoir.[7] Almost every cell type in normal circulation may be present: immune, mesenchymal, vascular, and nervous cells have all been identified in lipoaspirates.[2,7]

The adipocyte is derived from a connective tissue line of cells resembling fibroblasts.[8,9] Mesenchymal stem cells differentiate into spindle-shaped preadipocytes which increase their lipid droplet size, becoming more spherical, to develop into metabolically-active mature adipocytes.[8,9] The mature adipocyte consists of a single, large, central lipid droplet surrounded by a peripheral rim of cytoplasm containing a visible nucleus and other organelles, all encased in a thin external membrane.[9]

Adipocytes in subcutaneous fat are arranged into lobules supported by septa, a stroma of loose connective tissue, containing a dense capillary network. A high osmotic pressure gradient forces the cells into a tightly packed configuration within the lobule, each supported by a web of collagen fibers known as the extracellular matrix (ECM). The ECM, contiguous with the interlobular septa, connects each cell to the capillary network and also acts as a substrate for cell growth and proliferation.[4,7,9] This high capillary density, along

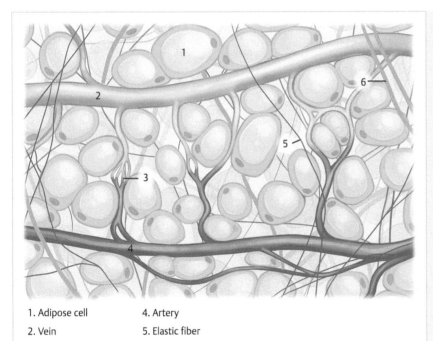

Fig. 2.2 Variety of cell types that comprise adipose tissue.

1. Adipose cell
2. Vein
3. Capillaries
4. Artery
5. Elastic fiber
6. Collagen fiber

with low O_2 demands, gives adipose has the highest partial oxygen tension of all organs.[10] The characteristic arrangement of adipose (cells compacted within rich microvasculature) and the high sensitivity of these capillaries to epinephrine allows for effective use of tumescent anesthesia and makes office-based liposuction a safe and bloodless operation.[4]

2.3 Physiology of Adipose Tissue

2.3.1 Functions of the Adipose Organ

Until recently, scientific belief resigned adipose tissue to the simplistic roles of energy storage, heat insulation, and organ cushioning only. This all changed with the discovery of leptin by Friedman and colleagues in 1994[8] a ground-breaking milestone which sparked an eruption of scientific interest and subsequent knowledge that continues to evolve to this day. Adipose is now considered the largest endocrine organ in the body[11] with known significant roles in lipid transport and synthesis, insulin sensitivity, and regulation of hemostasis, blood pressure, immune function, and angiogenesis.[8]

Energy homeostasis is an important function of the adipocyte, which is unique in its ability to store the most amount of calories in lipid form, readily available for rapid release.[8] At times of rest, adipocytes uptake circulating lipids (products of broken down ingested fat) and stored them as triacylglycerol droplets. When high metabolic demands increase sympathetic drive, adipocytes become stimulated via adrenergic receptors. This prompts hydrolysis of stored lipid and release of free fatty acids into the vasculature for use by other organs and tissues.[2,6,9] Perilipins on the surface of intracellular lipid droplets act as gatekeepers, preventing excessive hydrolysis. In obesity, perilipin concentrations decrease, rendering the adipocyte fragile and prone to free fatty acid release.[12]

Adipose also interplays with the endocrine system by releasing two hormones specific to and highly expressed in this tissue. Leptin exerts a direct effect on the hypothalamus, signaling satiety and decreasing food intake.[8,13] Homeostatic hormones, such as cytokines, insulin, glucocorticoid, sex hormones, and catecholamines, modulate leptin's release, thus implicating it in various other roles including glucose metabolism, human development, and blood pressure.[13]

Adiponectin is highly involved in the mechanism of insulin resistance by enhancing insulin sensitivity in muscle and the liver. It also promotes free fatty acid oxidation in tissues, thereby decreasing serum lipid concentration. In obesity, adipose maintains a constant inflammatory state, releasing cytokines that modify release of these hormones. Adiponectin decreases while leptin actually increases creating resistance in target cells. These alterations are implicated in the metabolic derangements and disease state associations (including atherosclerosis) associated with obesity.[12]

2.3.2 Adipose Tissue Development, Metabolism, and Turnover

Adipose development begins in infancy with cell proliferation. The number of adipocytes continues to increase through puberty before leveling off in adolescence and finally ceasing in adulthood. After this point, the total number of adipocytes in the body generally does not change. Lifelong obesity is therefore largely determined in childhood. Weight changes in adulthood generally result from adjustments in cell volume—hypertrophy and hypotrophy – rather than number.[2,10,14] Adipocyte number is tightly controlled in a constant remodeling process that carefully balances the rate of adipocyte apoptosis/necrosis with adipogenesis.[10]

Fat cell turnover begins with adipogenesis. The fully developed mature adipocyte averages 50–60 μm in diameter. Throughout its 10 year lifespan, the cell will continue to expand until reaching a maximum size governed by blood supply, about 150–160 μm. After this point, the cell will succumb to hypoxia and die. The dying adipocyte releases inflammatory factors that recruit M1 macrophages to surround the dying adipocyte, forming "crown-like structures", and phagocytose the lipid droplets remaining from dead cells.[2,10] These macrophages release more cytokines, in turn recruiting more cells and promoting angiogenesis and preadipocyte differentiation. In obesity, a higher rate of cell death overwhelms available resources and blunts fat turnover, precipitating accumulation of metabolically unfavorable fat over time.[10]

The commonly accepted "Lipostatic Hypothesis" explains the mechanism of body fat maintenance. Weight fluctuations trigger centrally-regulated autonomic systems that adjust food intake and metabolic rate until the set weight is regained.[10] Chronic energy imbalance can overwhelm lipostatic mechanisms resulting in significant weight change. Most patients seeking liposuction have unwanted fatty deposits amassed from a lifestyle favoring a positive energy balance state between diet and exercise. Adipocytes in this state will hypertrophy until a critical size is reached, about 170% of ideal cell size and determined by genetics and anatomic depot site. After this point, hyperplasia will begin.[2] Cells in obese tissue are generally larger, their size correlating with insulin insensitivity.[2]

In a state of negative energy balance, adipocyte size and volume reduces. Cells appear dramatically slimmed down with a paucity of lipid and increased adrenergic nerve fiber and vessel densities.[2] Glucagon and epinephrine activate triglyceride lipase in stored adipose tissue to mobilize fatty acids, resulting in weight loss.[4] This can vary by anatomic region: for example, in the gluteofemoral region of premenopausal region, there is decreased expression of adrenergic receptors with reduced lipolytic activity making this area is more resistant to weight loss.[2]

In the fed state, serum glucose increases activating insulin which antagonizes glucagon. With rising glucose levels, the insulin-to-glucagon ratio will eventually favor insulin. At this point, glucagon levels decrease and fat can no longer be mobilized. This raises important points about diet and nutrition. An ideal diet should both restrict caloric intake and promote stored fat mobilization. A diet rich in refined carbohydrates produces glucose surges, stimulating peaked release of insulin which inhibits adipocyte catabolism. Conversely, a diet of fats, proteins, and complex carbohydrates (i.e., fruits and vegetables), which require prolonged digestion and absorption times, maintains lower postprandial glucose levels, thereby effectively promoting weight loss (▶ Fig. 2.3).[4]

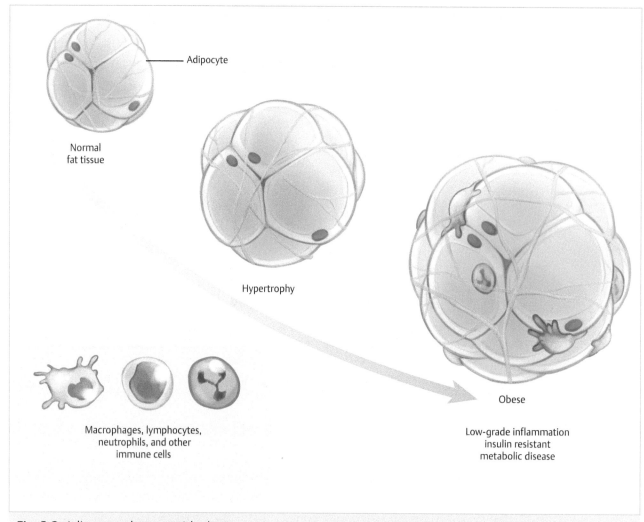

Normal
fat tissue

Adipocyte

Hypertrophy

Macrophages, lymphocytes,
neutrophils, and other
immune cells

Obese

Low-grade inflammation
insulin resistant
metabolic disease

Fig. 2.3 Adipocyte changes with obesity.

2.4 Biological Implications of Liposuction

2.4.1 Biological Effects on Cosmetic Outcome

Knowledge of lipostatic hypothesis begs us to question the implications of procedures like liposuction that reduce total body fat. While the current data are conflicting, it raises interesting points that should be included in preoperative conversations to ensure successful outcomes and manage expectations. Most lipectomy experiments have been conducted with animal models and generally show a compensatory increase in non-excised fat pads.[15] Similar results were seen in human studies which claimed that compensatory fat growth after lipectomy manifested as breast enlargement. This may have been due to general weight gain and body fat redistribution in non-aspirated areas, but alterations in the androgen-to-estrogen ratio could also be a contributing factor.[16]

A recent review summarizes data from human trials examining short- and long-term outcomes after liposuction. These results generally concur with the animal studies: postoperatively, patients experience an initial loss of fat mass and weight lasting up to 3 months. However, after 3 months body fat restoration gradually begins and is usually complete in one year.[16] Hernandez et al was first to evaluate anatomic fat redistribution in a prospective, randomized-controlled trial. Patients treated with liposuction of the thighs, hips, and/or abdomen were compared to an untreated control group. In the first 6 weeks, the treated group maintained a reduction in percent body fat and total fat mass. But over the next 6 months, the difference between the groups gradually decreased until none was seen at 1 year. Interestingly however, at 1 year, fat loss was actually retained in the thigh and hip regions while fat accumulated in abdominal regions, both visceral and subcutaneous, whether or not patients had actually received abdominal liposuction. Furthermore, the volume of visceral abdominal fat was significantly increased when compared both with postoperative volumes in the control group and with baseline volumes in the treated group.[16]

Several proposed mechanisms explain fat restoration after liposuction. Some theorize that cells injured by the liposuction cannula release inflammatory cytokines that promote adipogenesis.[4] Others suggest that the sudden shortage of stored energy triggers homeostatic mechanisms, inducing a compensatory adipogenic cascade. Based on this concept, Benetti et al investigated a strategy to improve long-term outcomes in a randomized-controlled trial. After undergoing abdominal liposuction, enrolled patients were assigned to either a training group, which maintained a vigorous thrice-weekly exercise schedule, or a non-training group. At 6 months, total fat mass decreased only in the training group, while visceral fat mass increased in the non-training group when compared both with baseline preoperative values in these patients and with results seen in the training group.[16] Thus, assurance of successful liposculpture outcomes is ultimately due to a combination of the surgeon's operation and the patient's dedication to appropriate diet and exercise routines to maintain a negative energy balance.

2.4.2 Metabolic Effects of Liposuction

While cosmetic outcomes of liposuction are clearly seen, much debate has focused around whether there are also metabolic effects. It is well established that a central (abdominal) fat distribution is associated with significant increase in risk for cardiovascular disease and type 2 diabetes mellitus, while a gluteofemoral distribution may actually be protective against cardiovascular disease.[1]

With this rationale, many have tested the hypothesis that surgical reduction of fat volume from certain anatomic regions may yield health benefits. However, results have been conflicting. A landmark study of obese patients undergoing large volume abdominal liposuction by Klein et al failed to show any significant differences after 10–12 weeks in multiple endpoints including insulin sensitivity and risk factors for coronary artery disease.[1,17] Others have reported similar findings in both obese and lean patients.[1]

Conversely, numerous other investigators suggest that significant health benefits do exist, especially in the obese population and after longer-term follow up. For example, Giugliano et al reported a decrease in insulin resistance and inflammatory cytokines with increased adiponectin and HDL in obese patients 6 months after large volume liposuction. Also noted was a correlation between the volume of fat liposuctioned and the degree of change in these factors.[1] Other studies, including one containing the largest reported cohort of obese women, showed not only similar improvements in insulin levels and sensitivity, but also decreased blood pressure and lipid levels, all at 3–4 months.

The reasons for such inconsistent results are unclear. One explanation may be that while most of the larger studies limited their treatment area to the abdomen, some smaller studies did not standardize treatment areas and included patients liposuctioned in multiple different regions. Only one study has examined patients undergoing liposuction to the gluteofemoral region alone. At 1 year, these patients maintained decreased fat in this region and also exhibited an increase in postprandial triglycerides, suggesting a detrimental effect of liposuction in this area. Other results further suggested that these metabolic derangements may be due to post-procedural mobilization of preexisting triglyceride stores.[1]

Although all of the above information suggests wide variability in cosmetic and metabolic outcomes after liposculpting, general patient satisfaction remains reassuring. In fact, one survey reported an 80% satisfaction rate after liposuction despite weight gain in 43% of responders.[16]

2.5 Biological Implications of Fat Grafting

Considering the biology of the adipocyte, a cell with fragile structure, high sensitivity to hypoxia, and adaptive propensity for cellular turnover, it is no surprise that fat grafting presents so many challenges. Reported graft resorption rates range from as low as 20% to as high as 90%. The commonly accepted "Cell Survival Theory" states that the success of fat grafting depends directly on the number of viable adipocytes transplanted.[18] Therefore, understanding the biological implications of the transplantation process can help surgeons to improve graft "take". The adipocyte's cellular structure (a large lipid droplet surrounded by a thin external membrane) makes it highly susceptible to rupture when introduced to the forces of negative and positive pressure and sheer stress during the process of fat grafting. Sheer stress during aspiration can be minimized by using larger cannulas (5 mm rather than 3 mm), which have been shown to improve viability and take.[18,19] High suction pressures and centrifugation speeds (up to 5,000 g) do not appear to have much effect on cell survival.[20] Many have studied the effects of stem cells, suggesting increased graft viability and take with a high stem cell concentration in the grafted tissue.[11] However, others report that tissue processing that achieves the highest possible concentration of pure fat for injection has the greatest impact on graft take.[21,22] Finally, sheer force generated during injection has been shown to significantly affect graft viability. Maintaining a low positive pressure by slow injection is most important, even more so than the diameter of the injection needle.

2.6 Conclusion

Once a highly underestimated tissue, adipose is now appreciated as a complex, dynamic organ. Recent discoveries have placed the adipose organ at the center of much scientific intrigue. Our understanding of its properties is constantly evolving with the proliferation of scientific data that continues today. With deep understanding and appreciation for the dynamics of adipose tissue, surgical outcomes can only improve.

References

[1] Pramyothin P, Karastergiou K. What can we learn from interventions that change fat distribution? Curr Obes Rep 2016; 5(2):271–281

[2] Cinti S. The adipose organ. In: Fantuzzi G, Mazzone T, eds. Nutrition and Health: Adipose tissue and Adipokines in Health and Disease. Totowa: Humana Press; 2007:319

[3] Markman B, Barton FE, Jr. Anatomy of the subcutaneous tissue of the trunk and lower extremity. Plast Reconstr Surg 1987;80(2):248–254

[4] Kaminski MV, Lopez de Vaughan RM. The anatomy and physiology metabolism/nutrition of subcutaneous fat. In: Shiffman MA, Giuseppe AD, eds. Liposuction Principles and Practice. Berlin: Springer; 2006: 1725

[5] Hoyos AE, Prendergast PM. Fat Anatomy, metabolism, and principles of grafting. In: Hoyos AE, Prendergast PM, eds. High Definition Body Sculpting. Berlin: Springer; 2014:8391

[6] Karastergiou K. The interplay between sex, ethnicity, and adipose tissue characteristics. Curr Obes Rep. 2015;4(2):269–278

[7] Tholpady SS, Llull R, Ogle RC, Rubin JP, Futrell JW, Katz AJ. Adipose tissue: stem cells and beyond. Clin Plast Surg 2006;33(1):55–62, vi

[8] Rosen ED, MacDougald OA. Adipocyte differentiation from the inside out. Nat Rev Mol Cell Biol 2006;7(12):885–896

[9] Slavin BG. The morphology of adipose tissue. In: Cryer A, Van RL, eds. New Perspectives in Adipose Tissue: Structure, Function and Development. London: Butterworths; 1985:2343

[10] Sun K, Kusminski CM, Scherer PE. Adipose tissue remodeling and obesity. J Clin Invest 2011;121(6):2094–2101

[11] Eto H, Suga H, Matsumoto D, et al. Characterization of structure and cellular components of aspirated and excised adipose tissue. Plast Reconstr Surg 2009; 124(4):1087–1097

[12] Greenberg AS, Obin MS. Obesity and the role of adipose tissue in inflammation and metabolism. Am J Clin Nutr 2006; 83(2):461S–465S

[13] Ahima RS, Flier JS. Adipose tissue as an endocrine organ. Trends Endocrinol Metab 2000; 11(8):327–332

[14] Spalding KL, Arner E, Westermark PO, et al. Dynamics of fat cell turnover in humans. Nature 2008;453(7196):783–787

[15] Mauer MM, Harris RB, Bartness TJ. The regulation of total body fat: lessons learned from lipectomy studies. Neurosci Biobehav Rev 2001;25(1):15–28

[16] Seretis K, Goulis DG, Koliakos G, Demiri E. Short- and long-term effects of abdominal lipectomy on weight and fat mass in females: a systematic review. Obes Surg 2015; 25(10):1950–1958

[17] Klein S, Fontana L, Young VL, et al. Absence of an effect of liposuction on insulin action and risk factors for coronary heart disease. N Engl J Med 2004;350(25):2549–2557

[18] Erdim M, Tezel E, Numanoglu A, Sav A. The effects of the size of liposuction cannula on adipocyte survival and the optimum temperature for fat graft storage: an experimental study. J Plast Reconstr Aesthet Surg 2009; 62(9):1210–1214

[19] Kirkham JC, Lee JH, Medina MA, III, McCormack MC, Randolph MA, Austen WG, Jr. The impact of liposuction cannula size on adipocyte viability. Ann Plast Surg 2012; 69(4):479–481

[20] Lee JH, Kirkham JC, McCormack MC, Nicholls AM, Randolph MA, Austen WG, Jr. The effect of pressure and shear on autologous fat grafting. Plast Reconstr Surg 2013;131(5): 1125–1136

[21] Salinas HM, Broelsch GF, Fernandes JR, et al. Comparative analysis of processing methods in fat grafting. Plast Reconstr Surg 2014;134(4):675–683

[22] Kurita M, Matsumoto D, Shigeura T, et al. Influences of centrifugation on cells and tissues in liposuction aspirates: optimized centrifugation for lipotransfer and cell isolation. Plast Reconstr Surg 2008;121(3):1033–1041, discussion 1042–1043

Section II

Noninvasive Body Contouring

3 Noninvasive Laser Body Contouring

John W. Decorato

Abstract

Body contouring remains one of the most popular cosmetic procedures. The advent of non-surgical body contouring options has led to a significant increase in the number of patients seeking a reduction in undesired fat deposits with an improvement in body contour. The noninvasive laser contour procedure is based upon the principles of tissue response to hyperthermia and the initiation of apoptosis with a subsequent immunologic response resulting in clearing of the damaged adipocytes. The 1064 nm laser wavelength was chosen due to its optical properties; i.e., depth of energy penetration into subcutaneous tissue with controlled heat deposition, lack of injury to overlying skin and potential for use in any skin type. Substantial fat reduction and lasting improvement in contour are noted following noninvasive laser treatment with the Cynosure SculpSure laser device.

Keywords: Noninvasive fat reduction, laser fat reduction, hyperthermia, laser tissue interaction, thermal conduction, apoptosis, 1060 nm wavelength

3.1 Introduction

Excess body fat is a significant problem in the U.S. Data collected by the CDC reports that approximately one-third of adults are overweight (BMI >25 and <30).[1] Body contouring, the removal of unwanted localized fat deposits, is a very popular cosmetic procedure. The American Society of Plastic Surgeons (ASPS) reported that over 635,000 procedures (both surgical and noninvasive) were performed in 2018 for the reduction of unwanted fat.[2] Liposuction, the surgical removal of localized subcutaneous fat deposits, is the most popular cosmetic surgical procedure performed.[2] Noninvasive body contouring procedures have entered the market as an alternative method of improving body contour without surgical intervention. According to ASPS, noninvasive fat reduction is now the 7th most requested non-surgical procedure.[2]

3.2 Hyperthermic Treatment

Tissue response to hyperthermia has been well researched. The studies of the effect of hyperthermic treatment on adipocytes demonstrated that a moderate rise in temperature of 5–10°C (42–47°C) will cause cellular and tissue injury by a variety of mechanisms including cell membrane permeability changes, denaturation of cellular proteins and inhibition of DNA synthesis and repair.[3] These injuries will result in delayed cell death or apoptosis.[4] Cellular and tissue injury will stimulate the body's innate and adaptive immune surveillance system resulting in clearance of the damaged adipocytes.

3.3 Laser Tissue Interaction

Lasers have been used in medical treatments for decades. The particular wavelength of laser light chosen for a treatment is dependent on the physical properties of the tissue and the absorption properties of the wavelength.

The energy absorbed by the tissue is converted into heat resulting in the controlled hyperthermia and subsequent injury to the targeted tissue.

SculpSure from Cynosure corporation is the first FDA approved externally applied device for laser fat reduction. The 1060 nm wavelength chosen for the noninvasive laser fat reduction device SculpSure was selected due to its optical properties in skin and fat. When compared to other visible or infrared wavelengths, 1060 nm is known to have minimal absorption in the skin making it a more efficient wavelength for delivering laser energy to the subcutaneous adipose tissue target without injury to the overlying skin.[5] This wavelength has a relatively higher penetration depth into subcutaneous adipose tissue, when compared to other wavelengths, facilitating spreading of the heat effect over a larger volume without creating a large temperature gradient or "hot spot" that may result in tissue necrosis rather than injury. Due to thermal conduction, the extent of the thermal effect in tissue from this treatment design is much deeper than optical penetration depth alone. Muscle and fascia, water-rich tissue, have a higher heat capacity than adipose tissue; therefore, the rise in temperature and potential injury is drastically less than in fat. The 1060 nm wavelength also has a low affinity for melanin allowing treatment of darker skin types, i.e., Fitzpatrick skin types V–VI, possible.

3.4 Tissue Response To Laser Treatment

Immediately after treatment, an inflammatory response is initiated. Ultrasound imaging of the treatment zone demonstrates evidence of an immediate inflammatory response with the appearance of a "cloud" (▶ Fig. 3.1). Within one week of treatment the response appears uniformly through the entire treatment area. Histological examination of the treatment area demonstrates lymphocyte infiltration within 2 weeks followed by invasion of macrophages resulting in phagocytosis of injured adipocytes with vacuole formation.

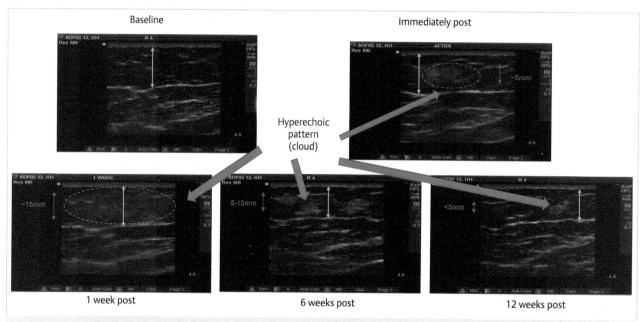

Fig. 3.1 Ultrasound examination. The inflammatory cloud that appears immediately after treatment rapidly spreads through the entire subcutaneous adipose tissue layer and gradually dissipates over the post-treatment time period. (These images are provided courtesy of John W. Decorato, MD, FACS.)

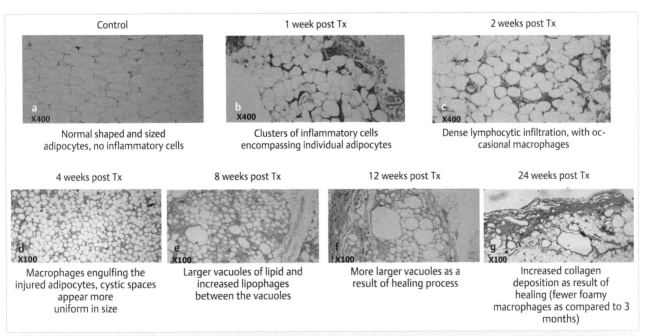

Fig. 3.2 Time frame of tissue response to a laser irradiation. (**a**) Control, normal shaped, and sized adipocytes with no inflammatory cells. (**b**) One-week post Tx, clusters of inflammation embracing individual adipocytes. (**c**) Two-week post Tx, dense lymphocytic infiltrate with occasional macrophages. (**d**) One-month post Tx, macrophages engulfing the injured adipocytes and cystic spaces appear more uniform in size. (**e**) Two months post Tx, larger vacuoles of lipid and increased lipophages between the vacuoles. (**f**) Three-month post Tx, more larger vacuoles as a result of the healing process. (**g**) Six-month post Tx, increased collagen deposition as a result of healing with fewer foamy macrophages when compares to 3 months post Tx. (These images are provided courtesy of John W. Decorato, MD, FACS.)

By 2–3 months after treatment, macrophages surround the adipocytes with significant reduction in adipose tissue volume (▶Fig. 3.2).[6]

3.5 Patient Selection

The SculpSure device is engineered to treat localized subcutaneous fat deposits. Establishing realistic expectations of the treatment is essential to patient satisfaction. The ideal candidate has a BMI of <30, and has "pinchable" subcutaneous fat. Visceral fat will not be adequately treated. Evaluation for treatment with SculpSure is similar to the evaluation prior to Liposuction. Standardized pre- and post- treatment photography is essential documentation for evaluation of treatment results. Although current FDA approval is for treatment of the abdomen, flanks, back, submental area and inner and outer thighs, off-label treatments include upper arms, calves, the suprapatellar region, "bra" fat and gynecomastia.

3.6 Technique

After marking the desired treatment area, laser array cradles are placed over the treatment site to permit maximum coverage of the region (▶Fig. 3.3). The laser cradles are secured in position using the adjustable belt system. Adequate "pillowing of the fat" into the laser cradle will ensure proper contact of the laser array with the tissue to be treated (see ▶Fig. 3.3). Lux lotion is applied to the skin to provide uniform contact between the skin and the laser

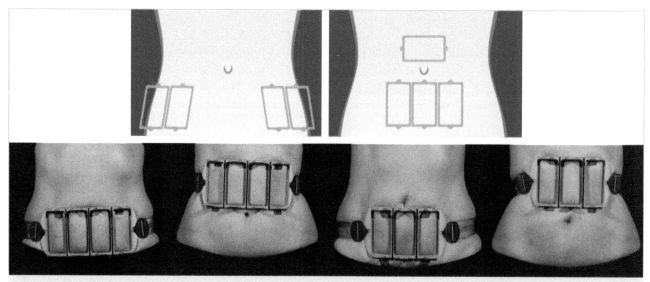

Fig. 3.3 Variations of laser array cradle placement. Note the "pillowing" of the treatment zone into the cradle to permit optimal contact between the laser array and the underlying skin. (These images are provided courtesy of Cynosure Corporation.)

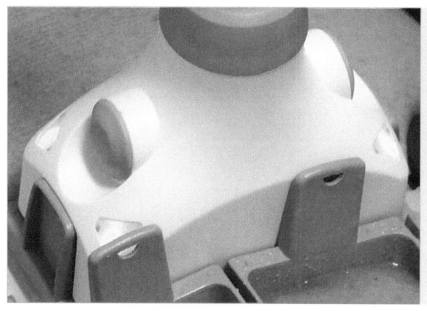

Fig. 3.4 Proper placement of the laser array into the cradle. Note all indicator lights on the array are green indicating adequate contact with the skin. The treatment will not proceed without adequate seating of the laser array into the cradle. (This image is provided courtesy of Cynosure Corporation.)

window. The laser array has a water-cooled sapphire window at the point of skin contact. Surface cooling provides additional patient comfort to the sensory nerve-rich skin during treatment as well as protection against superficial thermal injury.

SculpSure supplies 4 independent flat panels, non-suction laser arrays for placement into the cradle system. Independent power control for each array allows for tailoring the treatment to patient comfort and desired improvement. The laser array snaps into the cradle with an audible click. Once in proper position, a visible indicator light turns green allowing treatment to commence (▶ Fig. 3.4). If the array is not in proper contact with the treatment area, the treatment will abort. No laser safety eye protection is required as the laser will not function unless the proper contact between the laser array and the treatment area is established and maintained.

The laser was designed to create a smooth or even temperature gradient throughout the treatment zone resulting in a large volume of subcutaneous tissue heated to the therapeutic temperature range of 42–47°C. The maximum tolerable tissue temperature is limited by patient discomfort. Although power adjustability is possible, from 0.9–1.4 J/cm^2, high power settings are not mandatory to obtain the desired clinical effect. If the subcutaneous tissue temperature reaches our goal of >42°C and <48°C, clinically visible reduction in subcutaneous adipose tissue will occur over the ensuing months without evidence of tissue necrosis.[6]

The treatment is 25 minutes in length in 2 phases. The initial 4 minutes of the treatment is the "build" phase. This is preset to a power setting of 1.1 J/cm^2 although power setting adjustment is possible. During this period, laser energy is applied to the treatment zone to rapidly raise subcutaneous adipose tissue to the desired temperature range of 42–47°C. The 21-minute "sustain" phase of treatment involves the intermittent cycling of the laser on and off (laser duty cycle) to maintain the goal temperature range.[6] Adjustment in the power setting can be performed to the clinical endpoint of perceived heat within the treatment zone. Maximum power settings are not required to obtain clinical results from the treatment. This may result in patient discomfort limiting the tolerability of the treatment.

Following completion of the treatment, the laser arrays are removed from the cradles and cleaned. The cradle and belt system are removed. Little to no alteration in skin appearance is noted. The patient may resume normal activity. The use of compression garments is not necessary. Massage of the site may be of some benefit as tissue edema and temporary nodularity (fat edema) may be noted. If present, resolution of nodularity occurs within 2–3 months. Prolonged (>6 months) nodularity, while rare, may occur and is indicative of overtreatment with peak tissue temperature above 48°C. The treatments are very well tolerated without the need for pain medication. Side effects include, tenderness, swollen and mild discomfort that usually resolve within 2 weeks of treatment.

3.7 Results of Treatment

Clinical results of the treatment will become apparent at 6 weeks with optimal improvement at 12 weeks (see ▶ Fig. 3.7, ▶ Fig. 3.8, ▶ Fig. 3.9, ▶ Fig. 3.10, and ▶ Fig. 3.11) for patient before and after photos. In the initial clinical studies, patients underwent pre- and post-treatment ultrasound imaging to evaluate changes in fat thickness and pre- and post-treatment MRI examination to evaluate and calculate changes in fat volume of the treated area. Ultrasound imaging has been validated as means of measure fat reduction.[7,8,9] The images demonstrated a consistent and prolonged reduction in fat thickness in the treatment zone (▶ Fig. 3.5). MRI examination is a highly sensitive imaging test for soft tissue and volumetric evaluation is possible with reconstruction of the multiple slices taken through the treatment area.[9] The MRI demonstrated a 24% +/- 9% change in fat volume in the treatment zone (▶ Fig. 3.6).[6] These results were consistent throughout the initial investigative study and were later validated by Katz, Doherty, Bass, McDaniel, and Weiss in multicenter clinical trials.[10,11,12,13,14]

Careful analysis of the clinical trial patient treatment zones demonstrated reduction in adipose tissue beyond the actual treatment site. Follow up investigation demonstrated improvement up to 3 cm outside of the treatment zone.

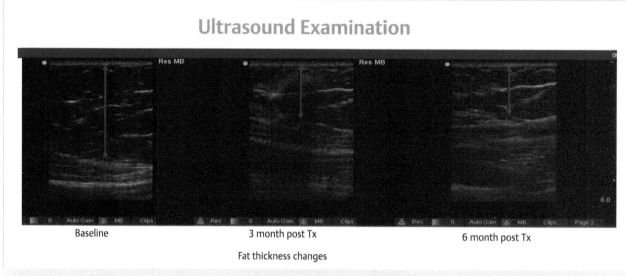

Ultrasound Examination

Baseline   3 month post Tx   6 month post Tx

Fat thickness changes

Fig. 3.5 Pre-treatment and 3 month post-treatment images following one treatment of the abdomen with the Cynosure noninvasive fat treatment system. (These images are provided courtesy of John W. Decorato, MD, FACS.)

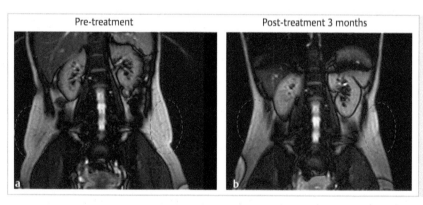

Pre-treatment   Post-treatment 3 months

Fig. 3.6 (a, b) MRI image of flank treatment zones pre and post treatment with the Cynosure noninvasive fat reduction system. (These images are provided courtesy of John W. Decorato, MD, FACS.)

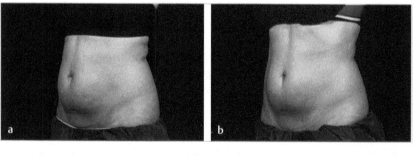

Fig. 3.7 (a, b) Pre-treatment and 12 week post-treatment images of a female patient who underwent treatment to the abdomen with the Cynosure noninvasive fat reduction system. (These images are provided courtesy of John W. Decorato, MD, FACS.)

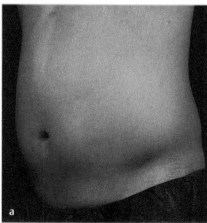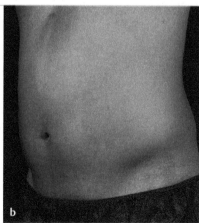

Fig. 3.8 (a, b) Pre-treatment and 12 week post-treatment images of a male patient who underwent 2 treatments to the abdomen and flanks with the Cynosure noninvasive fat reduction system. (These images are provided courtesy of Sean Doherty, MD.)

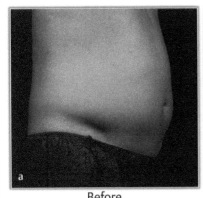 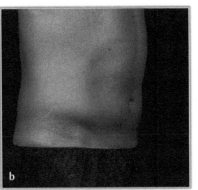

Before

12 weeks post Tx
weight change: -6lbs

Fig. 3.9 (**a, b**) Pre-treatment and 12 week post-treatment images of a male patient who underwent 2 treatments to the abdomen and flanks with the Cynosure noninvasive fat reduction system. (These images are provided courtesy of Sean Doherty, MD.)

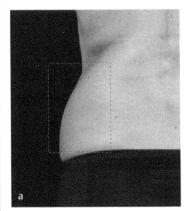 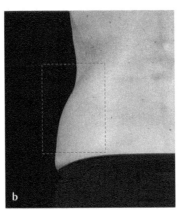

Before

1Tx; 12 weeks post SculpSure
Weight change: -2lbs

Fig. 3.10 (**a, b**) Pre-treatment and 12 week post-treatment photographs of a patient who underwent flank treatment with the Cynosure noninvasive fat treatment system. (These images are provided courtesy of Bruce Katz, MD.)

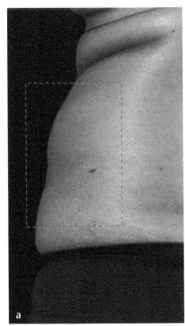 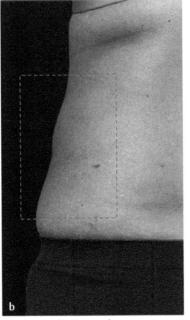

Before

1 tx; 12 weeks post
Weight change: −1lbs

Fig. 3.11 (**a, b**) Pre-treatment and 12 week post-treatment photographs of a patient who underwent flank treatment with the Cynosure noninvasive fat reduction system. The rectangular area is the laser array treatment zone. Note visible improvement in contour outside the treatment zone. (These images are provided courtesy of Bruce Katz, MD.)

This is theorized to be the result of the heat diffusion effect.[15] This results in a feathering effect beyond the treatment area and the absence of a distinct line of demarcation between treated and untreated areas. This effect may permit variations in cradle (and laser array) placement to obtain optimal treatment results.

Secondary treatment of the area may be performed at 6–12 weeks, with optimal clinical results with multiple treatments. Critical evaluation of clinical photographs of patients undergoing multiple treatments demonstrate greater improvement than the initial treatment. We currently theorize that the lymphocyte based adaptive immune response to the tissue injury results in an improved effectiveness of removal of injured adipocytes.

3.8 Limitations of Treatment

Although any patient with palpable subcutaneous fat can undergo treatment with SculpSure, a subset of patients was excluded from the treatment protocol. Any patient on immunosuppressive therapy was excluded from the clinical trials as lack of an adequate immune response to the tissue injury would likely limit effectiveness of treatment. We do not consider this an absolute contraindication to treatment, however based upon the necessity of an immune response to treatment, these patients may obtain sub-optimal results. NSAIDs were not considered a contraindication to treatment as these medications inhibit a different, non-cellular pathway in the inflammatory cascade.

Careful examination for hernias is necessary prior to treatment. Although temperature rise from absorption of laser energy is significantly lower in muscle and fascia than fat. Herniated omentum with its natural fat content may be affected by the treatment.

History of Herpes Zoster in the treatment zone requires careful consideration and prophylaxis with an antiviral agent such as Valcyclovir should be considered.

Treatment over open wounds is contraindicated as is treatment over fresh scars due to the potential for tethering to the underlying fascia and limited fat volume for treatment. Treatment over bony prominences is not recommended as heating of periosteum will result in significant patient discomfort.

Treatment over tattoos can be performed, however special care must be taken with respect to cradle placement and proper "pillowing of the fat" into the cradle. Inadequate contact between the laser array and the skin may result in additional superficial heat buildup. This may be due to metals, i.e., iron, present in tattoo ink. With proper skin contact and surface contact cooling, treatment over tattoos has been shown to be both safe and efficacious.

"Stacking of treatment," i.e., treating the same anatomic location twice during a single treatment session, is not recommended. During the investigative studies, it was noted that treatment for more than 30 minutes resulted in excessive tissue damage. The clinical result demonstrated nodular fat necrosis that did not resolve spontaneously.

Paradoxical fat hyperplasia is a poorly understood phenomenon which occurs after cyrolipolysis. The treatment area is noted to have an increase (hyperplasia) of adipocytes following treatment. This may be related to the role fat plays as an insulator in body temperature control. There is ongoing research into the etiology of this phenomenon. This occurrence, which may require surgical treatment, has not been associated with laser fat reduction.

3.9 Conclusion

The 1060 nm hyperthermic laser treatment is an effective method for noninvasive fat reduction. An excellent safety profile and high patient satisfaction an alternative to noninvasive surgical localized fat reduction techniques.

References

[1] CDC/NCHS. Health, United States, 2015. Data from the National Health and Nutrition Examination Survey (NHANES). https://www.cdc.gov/obesity

[2] 2018 Plastic Surgery Statistics Report. American Society of Plastic Surgery (ASPS). www.plasticsurgery.org

[3] Hildebrandt B, Wust P, Ahlers O, et al. The cellular and molecular basis of hyperthermia. Crit Rev Oncol Hematol 2002;43(1):33–56

[4] Nijhius E. Hyperthermia-induced apoptosis. Ph.D. thesis, University of Twente, Enschede, The Netherlands, 2008

[5] Decorato JW, Sierra R, Chen B. Clinical and histological evaluations of a 1060 nm laser device for noninvasive fat reduction. Paper presented at: 2014 Annual American Society of Lasers in Medicine and Surgery Conference; April 2–6; Phoenix, AZ

[6] Decorato JW, Chen B, Sierra R. Subcutaneous adipose tissue response to a noninvasive hyperthermic treatment using a 1060 nm laser. Laser Surgery Med 2017

[7] McDaniel D, Weiss R, Doherty S, et al. Ultrasound findings in fat following a 1060 nm noninvasive diode laser—correlation with anatomic findings. Paper presented at: 2016 Annual American Society for Lasers in Medicine and Surgery Conference; March 30–April 3; Boston, MA

[8] Barton FE Jr, Dauwe PB, Stone T, Newman E. How should results of nonsurgical subcutaneous fat removal be assessed? Accuracy of B-Mode Ultrasound. Plast Reconstr Surg 2016;138(4):624e–629e

[9] Chen B. Objective evaluation of fat reduction with a noninvasive 1060 nm diode laser. Paper presented at: 2015 Annual American Society of Lasers in Medicine and Surgery Conference; April 22–26, Kissimmee, FL

[10] Katz B. A multicenter study of the safety and efficacy of a noninvasive 1060 nm diode laser of fat reduction of the flanks. Paper presented at: 2015 Annual American Society of Lasers in Medicine and Surgery Conference; April 22–26, Kissimmee, FL

[11] Bass L, Doherty S. Noninvasive fat reduction of the abdomen: a multicenter study with a 1060 nm diode laser. Paper presented at: 2015 Annual American Society of Lasers in Medicine and Surgery Conference; April 22–26, Kissimmee, FL

[12] Katz B, Bass L, Doherty S. Objective evaluation of noninvasive fat reduction with a 1060 nm diode laser for treatment of the thighs and back. Paper presented at: Paper presented at: 2015 Annual American Society of Lasers in Medicine and Surgery Conference; April 22–26, Kissimmee, FL

[13] Weiss R, McDaniel D, Doherty S, et al. Clinical evaluation of fat reduction treatment of the flanks and abdomen with a noninvasive 1060 nm diode laser: a multicenter study. Paper presented at: 2016 Annual American Society for Lasers in Medicine and Surgery Conference; March 30–April 3; Boston, MA

[14] Bass L, Katz B, Doherty S. A Multicenter study of a noninvasive 1060 nm diode laser for fat reduction of the abdomen and flanks—6 month follow-up. Paper presented at: 2016 Annual American Society for Lasers in Medicine and Surgery Conference; March 30–April 3; Boston, MA

[15] Doherty S, Chen B. In-vivo and In-vitro tissue temperature during a noninvasive 1060 nm hyperthermic fat treatment. Eposter at: 2016 Annual American Society for Lasers in Medicine and Surgery Conference; March 30–April 3; Boston, MA

4 Ultrasound in Noninvasive Body Shaping

Jennifer Croix and Anne Chapas

Abstract

Focused ultrasound technologies offer methods for noninvasive fat reduction and body contouring that are generally safe, targeted, require no to minimal recovery time, and can be performed in office. These technologies act to ablate areas of subcutaneous adipose tissue (SAT) and provide a more permanent improvement compared to devices that provide temporary improvement by heating and tightening. Focused ultrasound technologies can be classified as high-intensity focused ultrasound (HIFU) or low-frequency non-thermal focused ultrasound and are FDA cleared for waist circumference reduction. Ideal candidates for HIFU and non-thermal focused ultrasound have >1.5 cm of abdominal subcutaneous adiposity and a BMI >30. Detailed treatment techniques for focused ultrasound treatments described in this chapter can yield expected waist circumference reduction by approximately 2–4 cm.

Keywords: Noninvasive body contouring, liposonix, ultrashape, high intensity focused ultrasound, low-frequency non-thermal focused ultrasound

> **Key Points**
>
> - High-intensity focused ultrasound (HIFU) and low-frequency non-thermal focused ultrasound ablate localized subcutaneous adipose tissue and provide noninvasive alternatives for body contouring with mild side effect profiles.
> - HIFU and non-thermal focused ultrasound are FDA cleared for waist circumference reduction.
> - Ideal candidates for HIFU and non-thermal focused ultrasound have >1.5 cm of abdominal subcutaneous adiposity and a BMI <30.
> - Based on current studies, expected waist circumference reduction by focused ultrasound is approximately 2–4 cm.

4.1 Introduction

Focused ultrasound technologies offer methods for noninvasive fat reduction and body contouring that are generally safe, targeted, require minimal to no recovery time, and can be performed in office. These technologies act to ablate areas of subcutaneous adipose tissue (SAT) and provide a more permanent improvement compared to devices that provide temporary improvement by heating and tightening. Focused ultrasound technologies can be classified as high-intensity focused ultrasound (HIFU) or low-frequency non-thermal focused ultrasound.

HIFU involves the delivery of high-frequency acoustic energy (2 MHz, >1,000 W/cm^2) to focal areas of SAT, resulting in a rapid increase of local adipose tissue temperatures to greater than 55°C, and subsequent coagulative necrosis in the targeted area. Additionally, negative acoustic pressure contributes to adipocyte destruction by disrupting cell membranes and inducing cavitation bubbles.[1,2] Microscopic examination of abdominoplasty specimens collected within hours of HIFU revealed a focal area of hemorrhage, disrupted adipocytes, interstitial edema, and coagulation of cells and intercellular collagen. These lesions showed a consistent size, expected depth, and no involvement of surrounding skin or fascia on gross exam.[3] Destruction of SAT stimulates a wound healing response with eventual removal of lipids and cell debris by macrophages from the treatment area and induction of fibroblasts. Significant damage to adipocytes with focal areas of fat necrosis and an inflammatory infiltrate are apparent on histologic analysis 4 weeks after HIFU treatment.[2] By 8 weeks, there is minimal inflammation, no fat necrosis, and lipid-filled vacuoles and foamy macrophages are observed. Thermal lesions are smaller, but remain apparent in the SAT on gross exam. Denaturation of collagen from the thermal effects of HIFU results in contraction and thickening of collagen fibers, which can be seen histologically and may produce skin tightening.[3,4] This effect does not occur with non-thermal focused ultrasound. Damage is limited to targeted areas of fat with no effects on surrounding tissues or overlying skin. Over 8–12 weeks the treatment zone is resorbed with about 95% resorbed by 18 weeks.[4]

Multiple studies have shown HIFU to be safe with most adverse effects being transient. Commonly reported adverse effects include mild to severe procedural and postprocedural pain and dysesthesia, mild to severe ecchymoses (▶Fig. 4.1), mild to moderate erythema, and edema, which are reported to last from days to up to 12 weeks.[3,4,5] Transient hard lumps, induration, and headache have also been reported. No significant changes in liver function, renal function, lipid levels, chemistry panels, coagulation studies, or blood cell counts have been reported to occur following HIFU when measured up to 24 weeks post-treatment.[5] There have been no reports of skin dimpling, burns, scars, or increased skin laxity.

There have been several studies evaluating the efficacy of HIFU for noninvasive body contouring. Fatemi reported an average waist circumference reduction of 4.7 cm 3 months after treating the abdomen and flanks of 282 subjects with 1 session and 2 passes of HIFU using 2 different focal depths of 1.1 to 1.6 cm and a mean energy of 137 J/cm². Lower energy levels achieved satisfactory results, but it was suggested that the minimum energy per pass should be 47 J/cm².[4] Fatemi and Kane conducted another uncontrolled, retrospective study in which 85 subjects underwent treatment of the abdomen and flanks with 1 session and 2 passes of HIFU at a depth of 1.1 to 1.6 cm and total energy dose

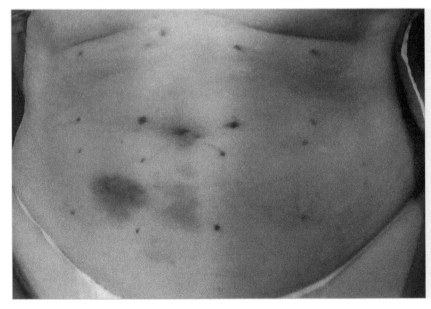

Fig. 4.1 Ecchymoses 7 days after 1 session of HIFU treatment.

of 104–148 J/cm^2 (average 134.8 J/cm^2). Treatment resulted in an average waist circumference reduction of 4.6 cm at 3 months after treatment compared to baseline. They similarly treated the abdomen of 40 subjects with a single session of HIFU, which produced a mean reduction in waist circumference of 2.9 cm at 3 months. Post hoc analysis indicated that there was no significant difference in waist circumference reduction when a total energy >133 J/cm^2 was used compared to a total energy ≤126 J/cm^2.[6] Jewell et al conducted a multicenter, randomized, sham-controlled, single-blind trial evaluating the effectiveness and safety of HIFU for waist circumference reduction. Subjects were randomized to receive total energy doses of 141 J/cm^2 (3 passes at 47 J/cm^2), 177 J/cm^2 (3 passes at 59 J/cm^2), or sham (3 passes at 0 J/cm^2) at a depth of 1.3 cm. Per protocol, both treatment groups showed a significantly greater average waist reduction compared to sham (-2.10 cm at 47 J/cm^2 and -2.52 cm at 59 J/cm^2 versus -1.21 cm for sham) at 12 weeks following treatment. Less pain was reported in the 47 J/cm^2 compared to the 59 J/cm^2 group.[7] Solish et al performed a postmarketing, single-blind prospective study of 45 subjects evaluating HIFU for abdominal adipose tissue without treatment of the flanks. Subjects were randomized to receive 3 passes at 47 J/cm^2 (total energy of 141 J/cm^2), 52 J/cm^2 (total energy of 156 J/cm^2), or 59 J/cm^2 (total energy of 177 J/cm^2) with each pass at a different depth (1.6, 1.3, and 1.1 cm). Waist circumference was significantly reduced at 12 weeks in all 3 groups with a mean reduction of 2.51 cm. There was no significant difference in waist reduction between the 3 groups, though a significant reduction from baseline was achieved more rapidly in the 59 J/cm^2 group. Additionally, the lowest energy group experienced the least discomfort.[8]

The effectiveness and tolerability of multiple HIFU treatment protocols for the abdomen and flanks, including different fluences (150 or 180 J/cm^2 total energy, 30 or 60 J/cm^2 per pass) and a grid repeat (passes) technique versus a site repeat (pulse stacked) technique, were examined by Robinson et al in an unblinded, randomized study with 188 subjects. Treatment resulted in a mean waist circumference reduction of 2.3 cm ± 2.9 cm at 12 weeks with no significant difference seen between the different treatment protocols. Patients in the 30 J/cm^2 groups reported significantly lower pain scores, again illustrating the advantage of using lower fluences.[9] Shek et al also noted lower fluences with more passes being associated with less discomfort in an uncontrolled single-center prospective study of 12 subjects treated with a single treatment of HIFU delivered at 30–55 J/cm^2 per pass (total energy 50–165 J/cm^2) based on the amount of pain experienced by the subject. Waist circumference was reduced by an average of 2.1 cm at 12 weeks after treatment with higher total energy, rather than the energy delivered per pass, being associated with greater improvement in waist circumference.[10]

The efficacy of HIFU compared to cryolipolysis for adipose tissue on the flanks was examined by Friedman et al Eight female patients were randomized to have adipose tissue on their flanks treated either by HIFU with energy doses of 140 to 160 J/cm^2 or cryolipolysis. There was no change in widest part waist circumference at 4 months, but both groups showed moderate improvement when scored by blinded investigators. There was no significant difference in improvement between the two groups. There was, however, a trend towards greater improvement with HIFU, suggesting that HIFU is at least as effective as cryolipolysis in treating flank adipose tissue.[11] There are no other studies directly comparing HIFU to other methods of body contouring.

In contrast to HIFU, low frequency, non-thermal focused ultrasound (200 kHz, 17.5 W/cm^2) leads to destruction of adipose tissue via mechanical disruption and cavitation without thermal effects at a depth of 1.5 cm. Using a porcine model, Brown et al demonstrated focal, well-defined cavitation of SAT with a length and diameter of 10 mm and 6 mm, respectively, and histologic evidence of adipocyte disruption with sparing of connective tissue, vessels, nerves, and overlying skin following treatment with non-thermal focused ultrasound.[12] The denaturation of collagen with subsequent contraction and thickening of collagen fibers seen in HIFU does not occur with non-thermal focused ultrasound due to the lack of thermal effects. Following disruption, adipocyte contents, primarily consisting of triglycerides, are released into the interstitial fluid, cleared by the lymphatic system, transported to the vascular system, and metabolized by the liver.

The safety of non-thermal focused ultrasound has been evaluated in multiple studies with side effects being transient and milder than side effects with HIFU. Reported side effects include transient mild procedural pain and dysesthesia, mild erythema, mild purpura, and blistering localized to treatment sites. No significant changes in laboratory tests including complete blood counts, chemistry panels, liver functions tests, or lipid panels have been observed[13,14] with the exception of increased triglycerides that remained within normal limits in one study.[13] Liver ultrasound has shown no steatosis. No nodules, skin textural irregularities, hypo- or hyperpigmentation have been reported in the treated areas.[13,14]

Studies examining the efficacy of non-thermal focused ultrasound for body contouring have demonstrated favorable results. Moreno-Moraga et al performed a prospective study with 30 healthy adults examining the use of non-thermal focused ultrasound on the abdomen (n = 10), inner (n = 2) and outer thighs (n = 10), flanks (n = 3), inner knees (n = 2), pseudo-gynecomastia (n = 3). Three treatments were performed at 1-month intervals. Circumference and fat thickness were measured via ultrasound 1 month after the last treatment. All areas treated showed a reduction in circumference with a mean circumference reduction of 3.95 ± 1.99 cm. The greatest reductions were observed in the outer thighs at 4.60 cm followed by the abdomen at 4.15 cm, though the differences between areas were not statistically significant. The mean fat reduction measured by ultrasound was 2.28 cm.[13] A multicenter, controlled study by Teitelbaum et al evaluated a single treatment of non-thermal focused ultrasound for abdomen, flanks, and thighs in 164 patients (137 treated, 27 controls). The mean circumference reduction was 1.9 cm at 12 weeks with no significant difference between treatment areas or between men and women. Fat thickness, measured by ultrasound, was reduced from baseline by 2.6 mm on day 14 and by 2.9 mm on day 28. The overall response rate was 82%.[14] Ascher investigated the efficacy and safety of shorter intervals for the abdominal region, performing 3 treatments 2 weeks apart on 25 female subjects. The mean reduction in waist circumference reduction at 112 days was 3.58 cm measured 2 cm below midline and 3.12 cm measured midline, suggesting the effectiveness of shorter intervals between treatments.[15] Hotta reported clinical outcomes for 70 patients treated with 1–3 treatments of non-thermal focused ultrasound on the thighs, flanks, and abdomen with an average circumference reduction of 2.5 cm per area.[16] Niwa et al performed a retrospective study of 120 subjects undergoing 1–3 sessions of treatment with non-thermal focused ultrasound. Treatment areas included the abdomen (n = 72), hips (n = 46), thighs (n = 30), dorsum (n = 1) and infragluteal region (n = 4). Mean reduction in circumference following 3 sessions for abdomen, hips, and thighs was 4.95 cm, 4.88 cm, and 3 cm, respectively. Infragluteal and dorsum regions only received a single treatment with mean circumference reduction of 2.35 cm and 2.6 cm, respectively.[17] Results of a multicenter, randomized, controlled study evaluating non-thermal focused ultrasound for noninvasive fat reduction have not been published to date. Details regarding the combined use of non-thermal focused ultrasound and other procedures are described later in this chapter.

4.2 Patient Selection

All patients should have a thorough history and physical exam prior to undergoing any focused ultrasound procedures. Patients with outright medical contraindications such as pregnancy, anticipated pregnancy, breastfeeding, emotional or psychological instability, and those seeking perfection should be excluded. Physical exam should include calculation of the body mass index (BMI) to rule out obesity, which is associated with visceral adiposity and diffuse subcutaneous fat. Patients should be overall healthy, have a BMI less than 30, and localized deposits of fat. For HIFU, patients must have at least 2.5 cm of adipose tissue. For non-thermal focused ultrasound, patients must have at least 1.5 cm of adipose tissue prior to strapping and at least 2.5 cm of adipose tissue after strapping. Patients with a history of keloid formation, poor wound healing, or chronic steroid or other immunosuppressive therapy should not undergo treatment. Patients with substantial cutaneous laxity due to rapid weight loss, pregnancy, severe photodamage, or advanced age, should undergo a skin tightening procedure concomitantly or prior to ultrasound treatment.[18] Abdominal wall hernias and diastasis should be ruled out prior to treatment as their presence may increase the risk of visceral damage. The treatment area should be devoid of large scars, wounds, abscesses, active skin disease, swelling, infection, inflammation, large skin folds, implants or foreign bodies (body piercing jewelry should be removed prior to treatment), or sensory loss or dysesthesia prior to performing a focused ultrasound-based procedure. Patients should not undergo a focused ultrasound body contouring procedure if they have had any of the following procedures within the past 90 days, injection lipolysis, abdominoplasty, surgery, laser, radiofrequency, cryolipolysis, or liposuction. For non-thermal focused ultrasound, it is recommended to wait at least 6 months following liposuction. For HIFU, patients should not be on medications which impeded coagulation or platelet aggregation. This is a relative contraindication for non-thermal focused ultrasound. Use of non-steroidal anti-inflammatory drugs (NSAIDs) for analgesia and daily low dose aspirin are permissible. For non-thermal focused ultrasound, patients should also be excluded from treatment if they have hypertension, ischemic or valvular heart disease, pacemaker, defibrillator, abdominal aortic aneurysm, hyperlipidemia, diabetes mellitus, hepatitis, liver disease, HIV, coagulopathy, bleeding disorder, autoimmune or connective tissue disorder, malignancy, unstable weight within the preceding 6 months, and abnormal kidney or liver function, coagulation studies, serum lipids, or blood counts within the preceding 3 months.[16,19]

4.3 Technique

4.3.1 Baseline Measurement and Assessments

Baseline photography, weight, and measurements should be performed prior to any ultrasound treatment for body contouring. Patient treatment areas should be photographed under standard conditions and body weight should be obtained. Thickness of adipose tissue in the treatment area can be assessed by manual pinch test of standard calibrated, spring loaded calipers and must be greater than or equal to 2.5 cm (1.5 cm prior to strapping and 2.5 cm after strapping for non-thermal focused ultrasound). Circumference measurement of the treatment area should be performed at 2–3 sites with a spring loaded measuring tape.

4.3.2 HIFU Procedure

Pre-treatment analgesia is prescribed at the discretion of the treating physician. Patients undergoing treatment at higher energy setting settings generally require pain management while patients undergoing lower treatment settings generally do not. Effective analgesia has been frequently achieved in our office with 60 mg of ketorolac intramuscularly 60 minutes prior to the procedure or 25–50 mg of meperidine intramuscularly 15 minutes prior to the procedure. The treatment area is marked with a 2.8 cm^2 grid while the patient is standing. Purified water is sprayed from the handpiece on the patient to couple the transducer to the skin for the efficient transmission of HIFU energy. The graphic user interface of the system console allows the operator to control the pattern of HIFU delivery in order to avoid bony areas or the umbilicus, thereby providing custom energy delivery that is unique to each patient's individual anatomy.

Energy delivery is tailored to achieve a total energy of 150–180 J/cm^2 in the individual treatment sites. Robinson et al demonstrated that the multiple different energy settings and pass delivery patterns can achieve circumferential waist reduction.[9] Energy can be delivered in a grid repeat pattern, where each site is treated sequentially a single time for full pass that is repeated multiple times or a single site can be treated multiple times in succession until the desired total fluence is delivered. Treatments performed at lower settings require more passes than treatments performed at higher settings regardless of the pattern delivery. Although all treatment levels can be effective as long as the total energy delivered is adequate, Robinson and colleagues found that higher fluence treatments trended toward greater improvements. In practice, we treat at the highest tolerated fluence until the total energy delivered is greater than 150 J/cm^2.

After the treatment, there are generally no specific postcare instructions for the treatment area but patients should be aware of expected side effects. Several reports have noted common side effects to be dysesthesia, ecchymoses, edema, erythema, post-treatment pain. These are generally mild to moderate and resolve within 2 weeks after the treatment.[7] Patients can generally resume all activities after the treatment and return for follow-up evaluation in 3 months after the procedure. Results 8 weeks following HIFU treatment in our office are shown in ► Fig. 4.2.

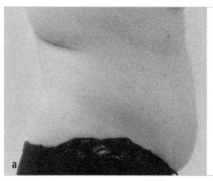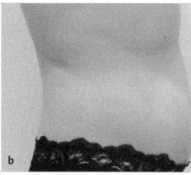

Fig. 4.2 (**a, b**) Baseline and 8 weeks following 1 session of HIFU treatment.

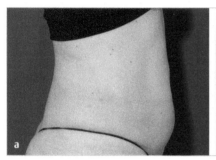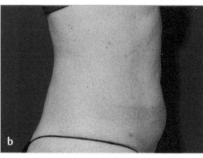

Fig. 4.3 (**a, b**) Baseline and 12 weeks following 3 sessions of non-thermal focused ultrasound treatment.

4.3.3 Low Frequency (Nonthermal) Focused Ultrasound Procedure

Patients should be instructed to shave any visible hair in the treatment area one day prior to treatment. Pre-treatment analgesia is not typically required. Areas of convexity are identified on the abdomen while the patient is standing and looking straight ahead. The treatment area should be at least four fingers below the sternum and be above the iliac crests. A reusable strap set is used to lift and gather adipose tissue into a central treatment area with the straps at least 5 cm from the lines marking the treatment area. The patient is placed in a supine position and blue drapes are placed horizontally at the level of the upper and lower straps. Three markers are placed in a triangular manner above and below the treatment area along the blue drapes to aid in camera calibration and tracking. After calibrating the camera, the treatment area is defined and scan mode (freestyle or guided) is selected. The freestyle mode, which allows user selection of treatment points, is fastest, but can result in inappropriate spacing of pulses. Ultrasonic gel is applied to the treatment area to couple the transducer to the patient's skin. The touch-screen control panel allows the operator to monitor and control the pattern of ultrasound delivery in the defined treatment area. Areas inappropriate for treatment or associated with discomfort, such as scars and bony prominences, may be skipped. The operator is notified once 100% of the treatment area has been treated. Three treatments are typically performed at 2 week intervals. Patients may resume normal activities following treatment, though a healthy diet and lifestyle are advised. Follow-up evaluation is at approximately 1 month with maximum results expected at 3 months. Results 12 weeks following non-thermal focused ultrasound treatment in our office are shown in ▶ Fig. 4.3.

4.4 Clinical Applications

Focused ultrasound treatments are intended for contouring of localized areas of SAT and circumference reduction. They are not meant for weight loss or treatment of visceral adipose tissue. HIFU is indicated in the United States for noninvasive waist circumference reduction, including the abdomen and flanks. In Canada and Europe, it is also indicated for use on the hips, buttocks, and thighs. Non-thermal focused ultrasound is currently only indicated for noninvasive waist circumference reduction.

4.5 Combination Treatments

There are no published reports of combination treatments with HIFU, but there are multiple studies describing the combination of RF with non-thermal focused ultrasound. The addition of RF increases the temperature of the adipose tissue before focused ultrasound application, which is thought to enhance the mechanical disruption of adipocytes by focused ultrasound. Chang et al treated the abdomens of 32 Asian subjects with vacuum-assisted bipolar RF for 5–10 minutes, followed by treatment with non-thermal focused ultrasound, and a second treatment with RF for 5–10 minutes to enhance lymphatic drainage, fat clearance, and aid skin tightening. A total of 3 treatments were performed at 2 week intervals. Waist circumference was significantly reduced by 3.91 cm and average fat reduction on MRI of two patients was 21.4% and 25% on the upper and lower abdomen, respectively. The combined procedure was overall safe and well-tolerated with no severe adverse side effects and only mild and tolerable discomfort in <9.5% of patients. Three self-limited adverse events occurred including allergic contact dermatitis to an adhesive band, transient mild erythema, and swelling and erythema leading to mild post-inflammatory hyperpigmentation.[20] Long-term effects of the treatment were evaluated 1 year later and demonstrated that positive results can be maintained at least for 1 year if patients maintain their body weight.[21]

Another study examining RF with non-thermal ultrasound for treatment of abdominal adiposity in Asian females was conducted by Shek et al. The treatment was divided into upper and lower abdomen. Each area was treated first with the radiofrequency device with pulse stacking until a temperature of 43°C was reached followed by immediate ultrasound treatment. Three treatments were performed every 2 weeks. Seventeen out of 20 subjects completed the treatment. Abdominal circumference and caliper measurement of fat were significantly improved at most time points with the median waist circumference being reduced by 2.5 cm at the 3 month follow-up. The procedure was well-tolerated with mean pain score of 2.3 and no severe adverse effects occurred. Six cases of wheal formation occurred after treatment which resolved within hours.[22]

It is important to note that there are no studies comparing non-thermal focused ultrasound alone to RF in combination with non-thermal focused ultrasound to determine whether RF had any added benefits. Waist circumference reduction with the combined treatments does not appear to be greater than that reported with non-thermal ultrasound alone.

4.6 Technology Pros and Cons

Advantages and disadvantages of HIFU and non-thermal focused ultrasound are summarized in ►Table 4.1.

Table 4.1 Advantages and disadvantages of HIFU and non-thermal focused ultrasound

	Advantages	Disadvantages	Timing
Both	Noninvasive Treatment focused to SAT No recovery time Performed in office	Must have >1.5 cm of SAT Not for visceral fat or patients with BMI >30	
HIFU	Tightening effect More controlled trials showing efficacy	Painful, can cause significant bruising	Single treatment
Non-thermal focused ultrasound	No to mild pain and other side effects mild and transient Has been combined with other body contouring modalities	No tightening Fewer controlled trials	3 treatments every 2 weeks

References

[1] Haar GT, Coussios C. High intensity focused ultrasound: physical principles and devices. Int J Hyperthermia 2007;23(2):89–104

[2] Shalom A, Wiser I, Brawer S, Azhari H. Safety and tolerability of a focused ultrasound device for treatment of adipose tissue in subjects undergoing abdominoplasty: a placebo-control pilot study. Dermatol Surg 2013;39(5):744–751

[3] Gadsden E, Aguilar MT, Smoller BR, Jewell ML. Evaluation of a novel high-intensity focused ultrasound device for ablating subcutaneous adipose tissue for noninvasive body contouring: safety studies in human volunteers. Aesthet Surg J 2011;31(4):401–410

[4] Fatemi A. High-intensity focused ultrasound effectively reduces adipose tissue. Semin Cutan Med Surg 2009;28(4):257–262

[5] Jewell ML, Weiss RA, Baxter RA, et al. Safety and tolerability of high-intensity focused ultrasonography for noninvasive body sculpting: 24-week data from a randomized, sham-controlled study. Aesthet Surg J 2012;32(7):868–876

[6] Fatemi A, Kane MA. High-intensity focused ultrasound effectively reduces waist circumference by ablating adipose tissue from the abdomen and flanks: a retrospective case series. Aesthetic Plast Surg 2010;34(5):577–582

[7] Jewell ML, Baxter RA, Cox SE, et al. Randomized sham-controlled trial to evaluate the safety and effectiveness of a high-intensity focused ultrasound device for noninvasive body sculpting. Plast Reconstr Surg 2011;128(1):253–262

[8] Solish N, Lin X, Axford-Gatley RA, Strangman NM, Kane M. A randomized, single-blind, postmarketing study of multiple energy levels of high-intensity focused ultrasound for noninvasive body sculpting. Dermatol Surg 2012;38(1):58–67

[9] Robinson DM, Kaminer MS, Baumann L, et al. High-intensity focused ultrasound for the reduction of subcutaneous adipose tissue using multiple treatment techniques. Dermatol Surg 2014;40(6):641–651

[10] Shek SY, Yeung CK, Chan JCY, Chan HHL. Efficacy of high-intensity focused ultrasonography for noninvasive body sculpting in Chinese patients. Lasers Surg Med 2014;46(4):263–269

[11] Friedmann DP, Mahoney L, Fabi SG, Goldman MP. A pilot prospective comparative trial of high-intensity focused ultrasound versus cryolipolysis for flank subcutaneous adipose tissue and review of the literature. Am J Cosmet Surg 2013;30(3):152–158

[12] Brown SA, Greenbaum L, Shtukmaster S, Zadok Y, Ben-Ezra S, Kushkuley L. Characterization of nonthermal focused ultrasound for noninvasive selective fat cell disruption (lysis): technical and preclinical assessment. Plast Reconstr Surg 2009;124(1):92–101

[13] Moreno-Moraga J, Valero-Alts T, Riquelme AM, Isarria-Marcosy MI, de la Torre JR. Body contouring by noninvasive transdermal focused ultrasound. Lasers Surg Med 2007;39(4):315–323

[14] Teitelbaum SA, Burns JL, Kubota J, et al. Noninvasive body contouring by focused ultrasound: safety and efficacy of the Contour I device in a multicenter, controlled, clinical study. Plast Reconstr Surg 2007;120(3):779–789, discussion 790

[15] Ascher B. Safety and efficacy of UltraShape Contour I treatments to improve the appearance of body contours: multiple treatments in shorter intervals. Aesthet Surg J 2010;30(2):217–224

[16] Hotta TA. Nonsurgical body contouring with focused ultrasound. Plast Surg Nurs 2010;30(2):77–82, quiz 83–84

[17] Niwa ABM, Shono M, Monaco P, et al. Experience in the use of focused ultrasound in the treatment of localized fat in 120 patients. Surg Cosmet Dermatol 2010;2:323–325

[18] Friedmann DP, Avram MM, Cohen SR, et al. An evaluation of the patient population for aesthetic treatments targeting abdominal subcutaneous adipose tissue. J Cosmet Dermatol 2014;13(2):119–124

[19] UltraShape Power System User Manual, Syneron, Inc.; 2016

[20] Chang SL, Huang YL, Lee MC, et al. Combination therapy of focused ultrasound and radio-frequency for noninvasive body contouring in Asians with MRI photographic documentation. Lasers Med Sci 2014;29(1):165–172

[21] Chang SL, Huang YL, Lee MC, et al. Long-term follow-up for noninvasive body contouring treatment in Asians. Lasers Med Sci 2016;31(2):283–287

[22] Shek SY, Yeung CK, Chan JC, Chan HH. The efficacy of a combination non-thermal focused ultrasound and radiofrequency device for noninvasive body contouring in Asians. Lasers Surg Med 2016;48(2):203–207

5 Three-dimensional Cryolipolysis Body Contouring

Villy Rodopoulou

Abstract

Three-dimensional (3D)-cryolipolysis is a safe and effective noninvasive technique for localized long-term fat reduction of all body areas, introducing a novel patented 3D technology and method. It is easily applied in a solitary hourly session with almost no recovery and is also providing an extra, almost regularly observed, tightening effect to the areas treated.

Keywords: 3D-cryolipolysis, freezing fat away procedure, noninvasive fat reduction, localized fat reduction, noninvasive full body contouring, skin tightening

---

Key Points

- 3D-cryolipolysis is among the best tolerated and effective noninvasive treatments for long term or even permanent reduction of medium sized fat areas in multiple areas of the body (abdomen, legs, flanks, arms, back, neck).
- The most common side effects are: erythema, swelling, bruising, numbness and slight discomfort.
- Results typically last for years and could be considered permanent, as 3D-cryolipolysis causes apoptosis to fat cells.
- The procedure is best combined with endermologie lipomassage for cellulitis improvement and bipolar radiofrequency or fractional for further skin tightening and tissue remodeling.

5.1 Introduction

According to the American Society of Plastic Surgeons statistics for 2018, while procedures like upper arm lifts and lower body lifts have shown substantial growth, for the first time since at least 2000, facelifts slipped out of the top 5 most-performed procedures last year, giving way to abdominoplasty (2018 plastic surgery procedural statistics from the American Society of Plastic Surgeons). Over the last few years the trend is growing toward noninvasive procedures. More patients are looking for a less invasive procedure that is effective in improving the body and face with minimal downtime. Under this context, cryolipolysis fulfills those requirements and is gradually becoming a favorite treatment for noninvasive body sculpting. According to Stevens et al the procedural growth was 823% from Jan 2010–2012 [n = 201 (2010), 671 (2011), 1857 (2012)] whereas Sasaki et al are stating that in 2014 more than 450,000 procedures were performed and cryolipolysis is becoming one of the most popular alternatives to liposuction for spot reduction of adipose tissue with high patient satisfaction rates.[1]

There are a number of other technologies available and their comparison of mechanism, pain level, side effects, and number of treatments needed are presented in (▶Table 5.1).

In 1970, Epstein and Oren coined the term "popsicle panniculitis" in their report, concerning the presence of a red indurated nodule followed by transient necrosis in the cheek of an infant who had been sucking on a popsicle,

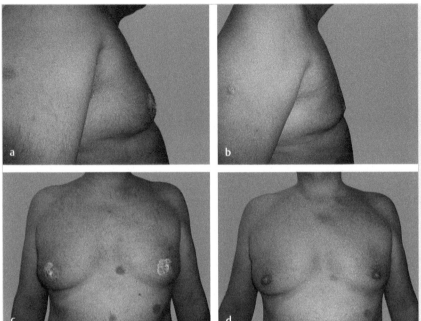

Fig. 5.1 Male, 42y old, BMI: 28, Weight change: + 2 kg, Post/tx: 2/12 following 1 session in breasts area (he also had tx on abdominal area and flanks with very good response). Skin fold fat caliper measurements: **(a, c)** BTx-R: 50 mm BTx-L: 48 mm **(b, d)** ATx-R: 30 ATx-L: 26. ATx-L: after treatment left side, ATx-R: after treatment right side, BTx-L: before treatment left side, BTx-R: before treatment right side.

Table 5.1 Comparison of technologies for fat reduction

Technology	Mechanism of action	Pain level	Side effects	Treatment needed
High-intensity focused ultrasound	Necrosis	High	Massive bruising and tenderness up to 2w	1–2
Unipolar radiofrequency	Apoptosis	Medium	Redness and tenderness 1–3d	2–3
Acoustic wave therapy	Apoptosis	None	None	8
3D-cryolipolysis	Apoptosis	Low	Numbness and bruising up to 7d	1–2
Low-level laser therapy	Apoptosis	None	None	6

Adapted from Cryolipolysis for noninvasive body contouring: Clincal efficacy and patient satisfaction. From Clinical, Cosmetic, and Investigation Dermatology, Dovepress.

and concluding that lipid-rich tissues are more susceptible to cold injury than the surrounding water-rich tissues.[2] But it was almost 40 years later that those observations were introduced by Manstein et al as a novel noninvasive method for fat reduction using freezing and given the new term cryolipolysis.[3] Although the exact mechanism of cryolipolysis is not completely proved as yet there are a few explanations of its function, like the induction of adipocytes crystallization, due to the vacuum suction with regulated heat extraction that impedes their blood flow. This cold ischemic injury to the targeted adipose tissue is further compounded by the ischemia reperfusion injury leading to the apoptosis of the adipose cells as well as to an intense inflammatory response, while the macrophages are executing the evacuation of the damaged cells and debris from the treated area within 3 months period.[4] However, multiple clinical studies showed no abnormality in serum lipid levels and liver function during and after cryolipolysis.[5,6,7] Also there is a transient decrease to the cutaneous sensation that returns to normal by 7 weeks after treatment with no permanent damage to nerves and skin of the treated area.[8] Moreover, there are studies that confirm its safety and efficacy over multiple treatments and in darker skin types.[9]

5.2 Patient Selection

- Women and men with BMI <30.
- Over 18 years of age.
- Presence of fat layers of thickness >20 (measurement using The FatTrack PRO DIGITAL Body Fat skinfold caliper) in body areas as neck, abdomen, hip rolls/flanks, brassiere rolls, arms, inner thighs, peritrochanteric areas, inner knees, ankles, male breasts, double chin, lateral neck.
- No weight change exceeding 5% of body weight in the preceding month.
- Agreement to maintain his/her weight (i.e., within 5%) by not making any major changes in diet or exercise routine during the conclusion of the treatment.
- May be candidates for liposuction but wish to try a noninvasive method.

5.3 Exclusion Criteria

- BMI <19.
- Under 18 years of age.
- Fat layers of thickness <20.
- Intra-abdominal fat or very fibrous fat.
- History of a fat reduction procedure (e.g., liposuction or other body contouring surgery, injection with fat dissolving agents, or other noninvasive procedure etc., the last year).
- Hernia or previous surgery on the intended treatment area.
- Any dermatological conditions or scars in the location of the treatment area that may interfere with the treatment or evaluation.
- Known history of autoimmune disease and/or malignancy.
- Known history of Raynaud's disease, or cryoglobulinemia, cold urticaria, or paroxysmal cold hemoglobinuria or any other known condition with a response to cold exposure that limits blood flow to the skin.
- History of bleeding disorder or if she/he is taking any medication that may increase the patient's risk of bruising significantly.
- Currently taking or has taken diet pills or weight control supplements within the past month.
- Active implanted device such as a pacemaker, defibrillator, titanium plates, or drug delivery system.
- Pregnancy or intention to pregnancy in the next 6 months.
- Lactation in the past 6 months.
- Unable or unwilling to comply with the requirements.

5.4 Technique

Our treatment protocol has been standardized following meticulous literature review as well as our experience with the, EC (European Conformity) marked as medical device, CLATUU (Classys Inc- Korea) on more than 550 patients and 3,500 hours/sessions of treatment the last 4 years with satisfactory results for more than 87% of patients following GAIS 5-point scale evaluation. This device comes with two pairs of wing shaped and flat applicators functioning with a particular, patented protected technology, which introduces a 360° surround cooling effect, contributing to a more natural and aesthetically pleasing result, avoiding irregularities. The amount of cooling (selected energy extraction rate) is controlled by the thermoelectric cooling cells powered by DC current and controlled by thermistors that monitor the skin temperature. Moreover, the latest model Clatuu Alpha is even more advanced and with multiple shape and size pairs of handpieces.

5.5 Evaluation-Consultation

Following a detailed patient history, the patient is examined in standing position and her/his intended treatment areas are evaluated for fat thickness/quality (fibrous or not), distribution and "geography" of the fatty areas, skin sagginess or existence of intra-abdominal fat. A first evaluation it can be done clinically using the "pinch test" and following that, using a skin fold fat caliper, with recorded precise measurements taken for future comparison between the same landmarked points according to the area treated (for example on the abdominal area: umbilicus-pubis, umbilicus-anterior superior iliac spine). According to the findings, the evaluation is explained to the patient including: the probable response percentage (it could be up to 40% with a mean of 25%), the time frame for the result to be achieved (approximately 3 months), the number of sessions that may be required, as well as the procedure itself and a plan organized in priority of the areas of more significance/problem. An approximate prediction for the number of sessions needed on the same area may be assessed. It has been noticed that if the fat caliper measurements are ranging between 49–59 the patient may need more than 2 sessions to achieve an optimum outcome, whereas if the results are in the range of 38 and 49 the patient may need 1–2 sessions. Usually one session is enough to treat fatty areas with less than 38.

5.6 Treatment

A tablet of paracetamol 500 mg is given to the patient orally about ½ hour before treatment.

Patient's weight is recorded and any change at each follow up visit to document results and ensure the patient is not gaining weight because of a poor diet or lack of exercise. Soft tissue deformities (unwanted fat deposits) should be evaluated from multiple views for best assessment. Following standardized photography of the areas the patient is marked in standing position in a similar way as for patients undergoing liposuction. The required skin pad, provided by the company as CLATUU Matrix Gel Pad, that includes the following ingredients: Propylene glycol, water, glycerin, phenoxyethanol, PEG-14M, sodium poly acrylate, ethylhexylglycerin, betaine, disodium EDTA is applied in order to fully cover the area to be treated and protect the skin. The application of the two available 3D-cryolipolysis vacuum applicators starts on the marked areas with few minutes of each other. According to the treatment areas selected, the flat or wing shaped applicators are used, always in maximum freezing capacity, but the suction may be applied gradually until the completion of the first five minutes in patients with low pain tolerance or in more sensitive areas such as arms, inner thighs or knees and in gynecomastia patients (where the nipples are pretreated with local anaesthetic cream and covered with selfadhesive dressing, e.g., tegaderm) (▶ Fig. 5.1). The flat applicators are usually used for the arms, back rolls, male breasts, inner knees, inner thighs, and ankles areas, whereas the wing (curved) shaped applicators could be used for the remaining areas. Particularly for the arms, as proposed by Wanitphakdeedecha R. et al, we position the applicator towards the lateral side of the arm to avoid entrapping the superficial aspect of the ulnar nerve within the vacuum applicator that is causing more intense pain and dysesthesia. Also, we advise patients to move their fingers continuously during treatment to experience less numbing sensation.[10]

Of course every patient and area to be treated are individualized and may need different applicator combinations and their careful placement and direction in order to avoid contour irregularities and undesirable outcomes and to achieve natural, aesthetically pleasing reduction of subcutaneous fat. Always the most prominent of the fatty area (bulge) has to be covered by the center of the applicator to become more affected by the 3D-cryolipolysis effect whereas the surrounding less prominent areas are less affected and a naturally "smoothed out" result is achieved.

The majority of the patients experience only numbness on the treatment areas after the first 5 minutes and can tolerate the 60-minute treatment cycle on each area very well. The same day up to two-three sessions in a total of four–six different areas may be applied safely and in the following days, more areas/sessions may be treated. However, in order to return to the same area for a second 3D-cryolipolysis treatment at least 10 weeks should have passed from the first one in order to consider that the result is final. According to Sasaki et al[4] there are three studies that assessed the theoretical enhanced efficacy with multiple treatments in the same anatomic area and demonstrated that a second successive course of 3D-cryolipolysis treatment led to further fat reduction.

Although a subsequent treatment leads to further fat reduction, the extent of improvement according to one study,[9] was not as dramatic as the first treatment and may also be related to the treatment area (abdomen was more responsive than flanks). This may be due to the level of the fat exposed to the second heat extraction which is closer to the muscle layer and its vascular supply may diminish the efficiency of the desired heat extraction or possibly that adipocytes that survived the first treatment have a higher tolerance to cold. Our experience is supportive of multiple treatments on the same anatomical area (up to three in certain patients) achieving additional improvement that leads to a more satisfactory final result (▶ Fig. 5.2 and ▶ Fig. 5.7).

5.7 Aftercare

Upon the end of the treatment the applicators are gently removed and 1 minute of vigorous kneading of the treated tissue between the thumb and fingers is applied followed by 1 minute of circular massage as described by Boey and Wasilenchuk.[11] They reported a significant improvement up to 68% within 2 months compared to the non-massaged treatment area. That may be due to the fact that manual massage is causing an additional mechanism of damage to the targeted adipose tissue immediately after treatment, perhaps from tissue-reperfusion injury. Sasaki et al also support massage post treatment application, with 5 minutes of posttreatment integrated preset mechanical massage using the device applicator.[12] It is advised for the massage to be performed

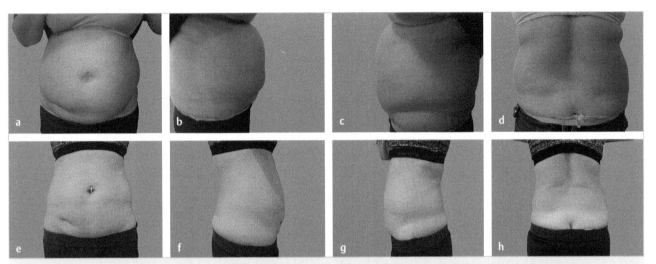

Fig. 5.2 Female, 43y old, BMI: 27, weight change: −5 kg post tx: 8/12 following more than 2 sessions in multiple areas of the upper body including, abdomen, flanks, back rolls, and axilla area demonstrating more than 50% decrease of skin fold fat caliper measurements. **(a–d)** BTx, **(e–h)** ATx.

with the patient still lying down as may be uncomfortable, and could rarely cause vasovagal reaction and hypotension. Nevertheless post-treatment manual massage is one technique that can be incorporated to safely improve treatment efficacy.

Also arnica cream for bruising prevention and bepanthol cream for quick skin recuperation from erythema are applied and the patient is able to return to their regular activities. The patient is advised to avoid sun until the erythema resolves but not earlier than a weeks' time and to return for a first assessment within one month's time. They are also informed that the treated areas may feel numb for the next few days (the longer observed period has been reported at three weeks) and to expect the final result in more than the 10 weeks' time. At that point, the patient may return for an evaluation in order to be determined if the desired result on the treated areas is achieved or if another session is needed. The most common complications following cryolipolysis, that generally resolve within a few days/weeks time, are: erythema, swelling, bruising, hyposensitivity, and pain. The temperatures induced in 3D-cryolipolysis have no permanent effect on the overlying dermis and epidermis consequently no permanent side effects have been described such as: scarring, paresthesias, blistering, hyper or hypopigmentation, ulcerations, or infections, provided that the machine and technique used are appropriate. There are some rare side effects described as the vasovagal reaction and paradoxical adipose hyperplasia that have an estimated incidence of 0.0051%, or approximately 1 in 20,000.[4] However none of those occurred to our patients until present time.

5.8 Clinical Applications

3D-cryolipolysis may be used in almost all areas of the body where fat bulges are found and they are more than 2 cm such as: abdomen (▶Fig. 5.3), back rolls/flanks (▶Fig. 5.4) double chin/lateral neck[13] (▶Fig. 5.5), arms (▶Fig. 5.6), inner thighs, peritrochanteric areas, inner knees (▶Fig. 5.7a), ankles (▶Fig. 5.8) and male breasts (▶Fig. 5.1). However, its FDA approved application areas, for the Coolsculpting System (by Zeltiq Aesthetics, Pleasanton, CA, USA) are until

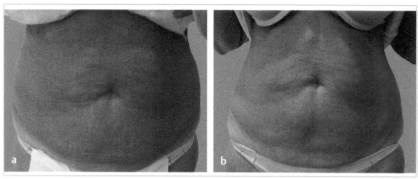

Fig. 5.3 Female, 66y old, BMI: 25, weight change: +1 kg post/tx: 1y following 1 session on abdominal area (she also had tx on flanks area with very good response as well). Skin fold fat caliper measurements: above umbilicus before Tx: 52 mm, after Tx: 27 mm, below umbilicus before Tx: 55 mm, after Tx: 29 mm **(a)** BTx **(b)** ATx.

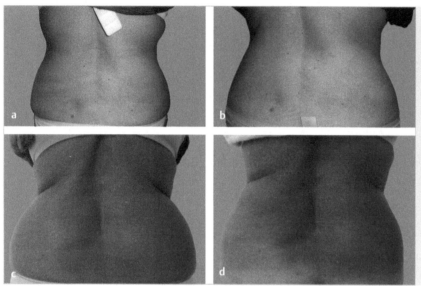

Fig. 5.4 Female, 42y old, BMI:22, weight change: −1 kg, post/tx: 2y following 1 session on flanks area and back rolls (she also had tx on lateral thighs with very good response). Skin fold fat caliper measurements on love handles: BTx-R: 51 mm, BTx-L: 53 mm **(a)**, ATx-R: 30 mm, ATx-L: 32 mm **(b)**. Female, 66y old, BMI: 25, weight change: +1 kg, post/tx: 1y. Skin fold caliper measurements: BTx-R: 58 mm, BTx-L: 59 mm **(c)**, ATx-R: 36 mm, ATx-L: 38 mm **(d)**.

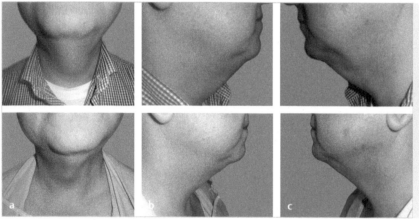

Fig. 5.5 Male, 51y old, BMI:27, weight change: −1 kg, post/tx: 6/12 following 1 session on submental/median and right and left lateral neck cryolipolysis area. Skin fold fat caliper measurements: **(a)** BTx-M: 24 mm, ATx-M: 17 mm **(b)** BTx-R: 20 mm, ATx-R: 14 mm **(c)** BTx-L: 17 mm, ATx-L: 12 mm.

now for the treatment of the flanks (2010), abdomen (2012), thighs (2014), and submental fat (2015) whereas it is used off-label to reduce fat in the back, arms, double chin and lateral neck, inner thighs, knees, lower legs and chest[13,14,15,16] (▶Fig. 5.9).

Special attention should be given to the abdominal area, especially in men, where usually there is coexisting intra-abdominal fat that cannot be addressed

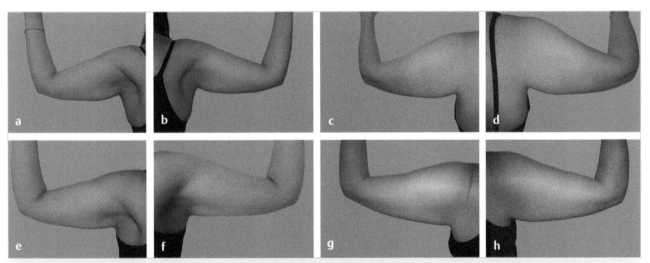

Fig. 5.6 Female, 37y old, BMI:25, weight change: 0 Kg, post/tx: 3/12 following 1 session on arms area (she also had tx on lateral thighs areas with very good response). Skin fold fat caliper measurements: (a–d) BTx-R: 25 mm, BTx-L: 30 mm (e–h) ATx-R: 17 mm, ATx-L: 14 mm.

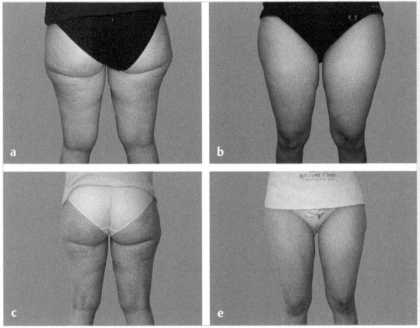

Fig. 5.7 (a–d) Female, 48y old, BMI: 21, weight change: –2 Kg, excessive skin sagginess post/tx: 8/12 following 1 session on upper legs multiple areas: inner thighs, inner knees, outer thighs demonstrating more than 40% decrease of skin fold fat caliper measurements (she also had tx on below flanks areas with very good response). Notice no deterioration but significant improvement of skin sagginess.

with the 3D-cryolipolysis treatment or even with liposuction and patients should be informed about it and have lower expectations (▶ Fig. 5.10). Another challenging area, due to coexisting or even predominating skin sagginess, are the arms in women and of course any area with skin laxity. However, there are studies that support cryolipolysis contribution in skin tightening.[13,17,18] According to Carruthers J., et al[17] the resulting skin firmness may be attributed to neocollagenesis stimulation. As dermal fillers may stimulate neocollagenesis by stretching of the fibroblasts, similarly the mechanical stretching mechanism due to vacuum suction of the fatty bulge may also be a contributing factor to neocollagenesis in cryolipolysis treatment and result to skin tightening. Our anecdotal observations as well have been quite supportive of that cryolipolysis "bonus" effect, clearly demonstrated on the patients with significant skin sagginess (▶ Fig. 5.11). It seems that 3D-cryolipolysis could be beneficial to the skin quality of the treated areas, in addition to diminishing

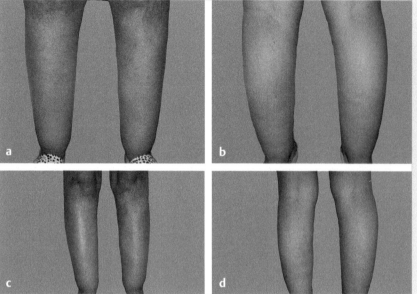

Fig. 5.8 Female, 53y old, BMI: 24, weight change: +1 kg, post/tx: 6/12 following 1 session on outer and inner lower legs (ankles area). She also had tx on inner knees with very good response. Skin fold fat caliper measurements: right outer side before Tx: 47 mm after Tx: 31 mm, right inner side before Tx: 53 mm, after Tx: 35 mm, left outer side before Tx: 51 mm, after Tx: 38 mm, left inner side before Tx: 55 mm, after Tx: 37 mm (**a, b**) BTx (**c, d**) ATx.

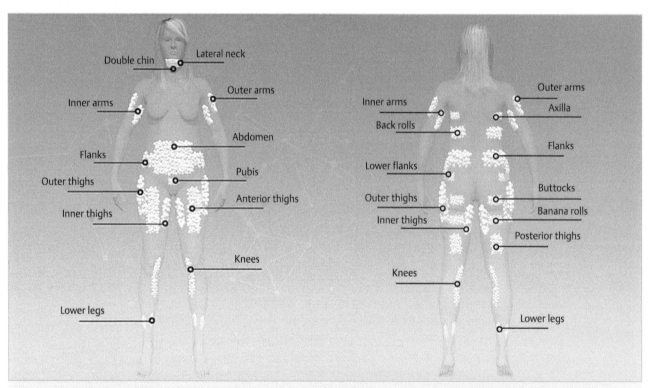

Fig. 5.9 Indications cleared by the US Food and Drug Administration and off-label indications for cryolipolysis as mentioned in peer-reviewed publications.

fat in the cryolipolysed areas. This could be attributed also to the very gradual fat destructive effect that 3D-cryolipolysis has, which allows the skin to adjust over time and without excess. Overall, this could be an important advantage of the technique for certain areas and for older patients with skin laxity; especially compared to classic liposuction where fat loss is immediate and the skin deflates almost instantly. Obviously, the cryolipolysis-induced skin tightening[13] effect that has been observed, provides another significant advantage of the method that should be investigated and elucidated with further clinical studies.

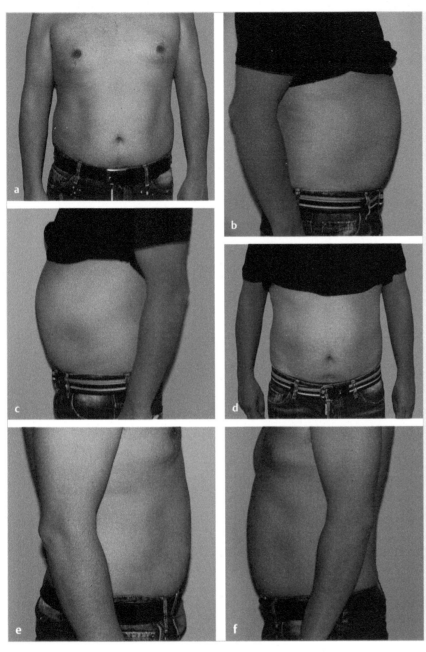

Fig. 5.10 Male, 42y old, BMI: 28, weight change: +1kg, Post/tx: 3/12 following 1 session on abdominal area Skin fold fat caliper measurements: Above umbilicus before Tx: 34 mm, after Tx: 18 mm, below umbilicus before Tx: 40 mm, after Tx: 20 mm **(a–c)** BTx, **(d–f)** ATx.

Finally, although all studies reported a fat reduction in every area examined it is not yet clarified which areas are the most responsive to 3D-cryolipolysis and what are the favorable characteristics for an optimal result (e.g., fat depots vascularity, metabolic activity, or location). It has been observed that fibrous fat is more difficult to treat, probably because it is harder to be suctioned into the vacuum applicator and has more interlobular connections between the adipose lobular cells to be destructed. As a result, it may require more sessions than the malleable fat. Patients and doctors should be aware of this, during consultation and may need to be treat these areas using a conformable-surface applicators that are available in variant shapes and sizes.[14]

While 3D-cryolipolysis is reducing (presumably permanently) fat cells, endermologie is completing the result by diminishing the remaining superficial fibrous connections, that are causing the characteristic 'orange skin' look, and is also assisting to the faster lymphatic drainage. It could be quite

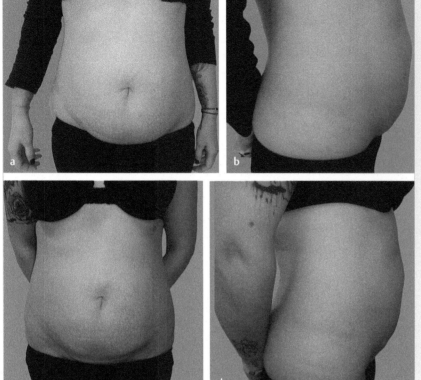

Fig. 5.11 Female, 31y old, BMI: 22, weight change: −1 Kg, coexisting excessive skin sagginess with prominent striae post/tx: 4/12 following 1 session on abdominal area. Notice no deterioration but significant improvement of skin firmness. Skin fold fat caliper measurements: above umbilicus before Tx: 53 mm, after Tx: 39 mm, below umbilicus before Tx: 44 mm, after Tx: 35 mm **(a, b)** BTx **(c, d)** ATx.

helpful as a pre- as well as-post 3D-cryolipolysis treatment. A combination of tailor-made treatments could be formed according to each patient's needs. Also 3D-cryolipolysis could be combined with skin tightening treatments using bipolar or monopolar radiofrequency systems. Radiofrequency treatments could provide more of a tightening effect beyond what 3D-cryolipolysis seems to offer as well as improvement in skin apperance. There are a few devices available on the market, either monopolar devices like Accent Prime (Alma Lasers) which is combined with ultrasound, or bipolar radiofrequency such as, the FDA approved VelaShape III–for cellulitis treatment (Candela). Moreover, the BodyFX, the MiniFX and the Plus are all quite strong bipolar radiofrequency handpieces (InMode Aesthetic Solutions) that could result to long term cellulite and body contouring improvements.[19] Recently, a new and effective modality was approved by the FDA, the Morpheus8 (InMode Aesthetic Solutions)[20] which is a microneedling device that utilizes radiofrequency energy to remodel and contour the face and body via subdermal adipose remodeling. Ideally these treatments may be scheduled a few days following the 3D-cryolipolysis session in order to provide an optimal result, especially in areas with coexisting skin saginess and/or skin surface abnormalities.

References

[1] Stevens WG, Pietrzak LK, Spring MA. Broad overview of a clinical and commercial experience with CoolSculpting. Aesthet Surg J 2013; 33(6):835–846

[2] Epstein EH, Jr, Oren ME. Popsicle panniculitis. N Engl J Med 1970; 282(17):966–967

[3] Manstein D, Laubach H, Watanabe K, Farinelli W, Zurakowski D, Anderson RR. Selective cryolysis: a novel method of noninvasive fat removal. Lasers Surg Med 2008; 40(9):595–604

[4] Ingargiola MJ, Motakef S, Chung MT, Vasconez HC, Sasaki GH. Cryolipolysis for fat reduction and body contouring: safety and efficacy of current treatment paradigms. Plast Reconstr Surg 2015; 135(6):1581–1590

[5] Ferraro GA, De Francesco F, Cataldo C, Rossano F, Nicoletti G, D'Andrea F. Synergistic effects of cryolipolysis and shock waves for noninvasive body contouring. Aesthetic Plast Surg 2012; 36(3):666–679

[6] Lee KR. Clinical efficacy of fat reduction on the thigh of Korean women through cryolipolysis. J Obes Weight Loss Ther 2013; 3:1–5

[7] Riopelle JT, Kovach B. Lipid and liver function effects of the cryolipolysis procedure in a study of male love handle reduction. Lasers Surg Med 2009;82

[8] Coleman SR, Sachdeva K, Egbert BM, Preciado J, Allison J. Clinical efficacy of noninvasive cryolipolysis and its effects on peripheral nerves. Aesthetic Plast Surg 2009; 33(4):482–488

[9] Shek SY, Chan NP, Chan HH. Noninvasive cryolipolysis for body contouring in Chinese--a first commercial experience. Lasers Surg Med 2012; 44(2):125–130

[10] Wanitphakdeedecha R, Sathaworawong A, Manuskiatti W. The efficacy of cryolipolysis treatment on arms and inner thighs. Lasers Med Sci 2015; 30(8):2165–2169

[11] Boey GE, Wasilenchuk JL. Enhanced clinical outcome with manual massage following cryolipolysis treatment: a 4-month study of safety and efficacy. Lasers Surg Med 2014; 46(1):20–26

[12] Sasaki GH, Abelev N, Tevez-Ortiz A. Noninvasive Selective Cryolipolysis and Reperfusion Recovery for Localized Natural Fat Reduction and Contouring. Aesthetic Surgery Journal 2014; 34(3):420–431

[13] Rodopoulou S, Gavala M-I, Keramidas E. Three-dimensional cryolipolysis for submental and lateral neck fat reduction. Plast Reconstr surgery Glob open. 2020;8(4):e2789. doi:10.1097/GOX.0000000000002789

[14] Stevens WG, Bachelor EP. Cryolipolysis conformable-surface applicator for nonsurgical fat reduction in lateral thighs. Aesthet Surg J 2015; 35(1):66–71

[15] Zelickson BD, Burns AJ, Kilmer SL. Cryolipolysis for safe and effective inner thigh fat reduction. Lasers Surg Med 2015; 47(2):120–127

[16] Kilmer SL, Burns AJ, Zelickson BD. Safety and efficacy of cryolipolysis for noninvasive reduction of submental fat. Lasers Surg Med 2016; 48(1):3–13

[17] Carruthers J, Stevens WG, Carruthers A, Humphrey S. Cryolipolysis and skin tightening. Dermatol Surg 2014; 40(Suppl 12):S184–S189

[18] Stevens WG. Does Cryolipolysis Lead to Skin Tightening? A First Report of Cryodermadstringo. Aesthet Surg J 2014; 34(6):NP32–NP34

[19] Mulholland RS, Paul MD, Chalfoun C. Noninvasive body contouring with radiofrequency, ultrasound, cryolipolysis, and low-level laser therapy. Clin Plast Surg 2011; 38(3):503–520, vii–iii

[20] Dayan E, Chia C, Burns AJ, Theodorou S. Adjustable depth fractional radiofrequency combined with bipolar radiofrequency: a minimally invasive combination treatment for skin laxity. Aesthet Surg J. 2019;39(Suppl_3):S112-S119. doi:10.1093/asj/sjz055

6 Noninvasive Radiofrequency Fat Destruction for Body Contouring

Alix O'Brien and Sherrell J. Aston

Abstract

Selective noninvasive radiofrequency fat destruction for body contouring using the BTL Vanquish ME (maximum energy) produces some permanent destruction of subcutaneous fat cells. Four to six 45-minute treatment sessions by a non-contact application for each body part area (abdomen, love handles, thighs) are usually advised. Some improvement of the results with radiofrequency fat destruction will continue to become more obvious by 3–4 months. While the results are moderate when compared to liposuction, patients like the non-surgical treatment with no down time.

Keywords: Radiofrequency, fat destruction, body contouring, BTL Vanquish

BTL Vanquish ME has quickly risen to the top of the "non-surgical device" chain by providing circumferential reduction of the abdomen with no anesthesia, pain, or down time. BTL Vanquish ME is a selective radiofrequency device that targets subcutaneous adipose tissue, permanently reducing the number of fat cells in the area treated. During treatment, the unit's non-contact device (or applicator) is positioned over the area to be treated and delivers RF-based energy, initiating induced apoptosis in the fat layers.[1] The treatment protocol recommends four weekly sessions of 45 minute duration to achieve results. It takes approximately 21 days for the absorption and excretion of the destroyed adipose cells to occur, so one can expect to see full results 3 to 4 weeks after their final treatment. We have found that six treatments improve results significantly and offer up to twice weekly sessions if hydration levels are maintained—a crucial component to a successful Vanquish ME series.

Long before radiofrequency devices were used in the aesthetic arena they were used in other areas of medicine such as pain management. BTL, a leading manufacturer of both medical and aesthetic devices, was founded in 1993 in Prague, Czech Republic. The company's early years were devoted to the development and advancement of devices which used targeted radiofrequency therapy to treat pain. The discovery that such technology might also destroy fat cells led to the research and development of the aesthetic devices we use today. A 2013 study using Vietnamese pigs led to the following conclusion, "A new model of fat reduction using high-frequency RF has been successfully achieved in a porcine model. This has very positive implications in the development of an operator independent, contact free device for reduction of fat in clinical practice."[2] In 2013, BTL introduced Vanquish, a non-surgical fat reduction device unlike any others on the market due to its non-contact, large spot size applicator and painless treatments. Using a patented Energy Flow Control (EFC) system, this device automatically tunes the tissue-applicator-generator circuitry to selectively deliver the energy to the adipose tissue layer while minimizing the risk of overheating of the skin, muscles, or internal organs.[3] The original Vanquish has since been upgraded to the Vanquish ME system we currently use today. The new system provides the patient with more targeted heat and does so more efficiently than the original device. BTL Vanquish ME offers improved tuning performance, more concentrated thermal energy and less scatter to non-fatty tissue.[4] We have found the results with the upgraded system to be superior and the treatments still tolerable, but hotter than what was felt with the original device.

A common question asked during fat reduction consultations is how BTL Vanquish ME can heat the subcutaneous fat to a degree that initiates induced apoptosis without causing thermal injury to the skin, muscle, and deeper structures. Skin and muscle tissue contain a significant amount of water while fat does not. Radiofrequency waves travel easily through water and therefore penetrate the skin quickly, but are unable to get past the subcutaneous fat layer. Only when impeded in the subcutaneous fat layer does the energy heat to apoptotic temperature levels. The energy is essentially trapped in the fat layer leaving minimal risk to the muscle and deeper structures (▶Fig. 6.1). Patients feel what has been described as "a comfortable warmth" and often times find the treatment pleasurable. The combination of the skin temperature remaining at a lower degree than the adipose tissue and the device's multiple skin cooling features contribute to patient comfort during treatment.

It is an absolute necessity for patients to be well-hydrated during treatments with BTL Vanquish ME. Well-hydrated skin allows more energy to penetrate the skin and impede the fat layer inducing greater apoptosis. Patients should increase their water consumption beginning the day before a treatment, and continue hydrating the day of, and day following a Vanquish ME session. The following hydration recommendation was made in The Supplement to Modern Aesthetic Journal, "Patients who are well-hydrated rapidly reach 200 watts of energy, while those who are not well-hydrated may not reach this desired energy peak. To encourage rapid and high-energy attainment, instruct patients to drink half their body weight in ounces the day of, the day before, and the day after Vanquish ME treatment."[5]

Vanquish ME is most effective in treating diet and exercise resistant areas of fat in individuals otherwise at a healthy weight. The initial consultation will determine if a patient is a good candidate for Vanquish ME. Although Vanquish ME is not designed to be a weight loss procedure, it is a good tool to "jump start" a patient's weight loss effort. Patients are motivated by results and seeing a positive change from Vanquish ME inspires people to make the lifestyle changes associated with long term weight loss. The amount of change is variable, however anyone with excess subcutaneous fat treated with Vanquish ME will see a result (▶Fig. 6.2). According to Dr. Jerry L. Cooper, "Treatment is

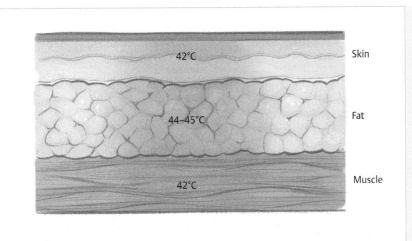

Fig. 6.1 Apoptic temperature levels.

42°C — Skin

44–45°C — Fat

42°C — Muscle

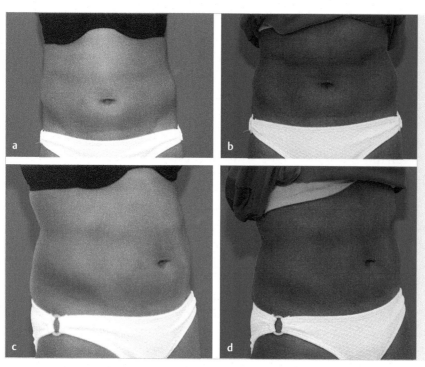

Fig. 6.2 (a–d) Before and one month after photographs of a series of 4 Vanquish treatments to the abdomen.

appropriate for any patient with external fat-fat that can be pinched between the thumb and index finger."[5] It is often times offered as a non-surgical alternative for people who would benefit from liposuction but do not want to have a surgical procedure, or in whom surgery is contraindicated. Unlike many non-surgical devices, Vanquish ME can treat all skin types and has zero downtime. Patients can go right back to work after treatment and are encouraged to exercise in the days following. The most common areas treated are the abdomen (upper and lower), love handles, and "bra fat". The large, non-contact applicator has side panels which allow for additional contouring to the waist when treating the abdomen or back. The abdomen can often times be treated as a single area, however if the area of excess fat is both superior and inferior to the umbilicus in a patient with a long torso it is necessary to treat it as two areas.

There are different ways to approach a patient who has multiple areas of concern. In most patients each area is treated individually with a series of six treatments, completing one series before beginning the next. We have found that this allows patients to assess their results before investing more time and money into additional areas. We know they are going to get a result, however, a patient's true expectation of a result can only be determined after the fact and we ultimately want people to feel like their return on financial investment was worth it. In addition to giving people the opportunity to weigh the cost/benefit ratio it can be difficult for patients to lie still for the hour and a half it takes to treat two areas consecutively. There is additional time needed to reposition the patient from supine to prone (or vice versa) and set up the device a second time. On occasion if a patient is most concerned with their abdomen, but has minor bulging of the love handles, a hybrid treatment of forty-five minutes to the abdomen, and fifteen minutes to the love handles will be done to optimize the circumferential reduction. It is well worth adding the additional time at no additional cost to enhance the result and have a happy patient in the end. Patients are typically treated with Vanquish ME once a week for 6 weeks, however patients that are able to stay well-hydrated and are looking for expedited results can do twice-weekly sessions. There are exceptions with people feeling and seeing changes sooner, but most patients can expect to see their full result about a month after their last treatment. It should be noted that BTL Vanquish ME is contraindicated in people with metal implants and any active implanted medical device.

BTL Vanquish ME is as close to a "one size fits" all device you can come by for fat reduction. It can be used on all skin types, treats the smallest area of excess fat to bulk reduction, and is very popular among both men and women. More and more men are embracing cosmetic procedures to improve their appearance and this trend will continue to rise. The growing number of non-surgical options is a contributing factor to the increase in male patients. This is beneficial for BTL Vanquish ME since so many men have excess fat in their abdomen, love handles, and flanks. Even more so than women, men like to be discreet about having cosmetic procedures and are turned off by the idea of pain and/or downtime from a procedure. Since bringing the original Vanquish into the practice we have seen an influx of men who otherwise might not have come through the front door. Some of these men have been determined to be better liposuction candidates and have gone on to have surgery. Others opted for non-surgical radiofrequency treatments to either avoid surgery or because their excess fat was minimal. Having more options for patients has proven to be appealing to patients and financially beneficial to the practice. Most men and women find Vanquish ME to be a comfortable experience, feeling heat but not overheated, with the "rare hot" spot easily alleviated by moving the device or lowering the wattage.

During a treatment the patient lies underneath the device's large spot, non-contact applicator which attaches to an "arm" that is designed to optimally position the applicator (▶ Fig. 6.3). The official recommendation is for the applicator to be positioned 10mm away from the skin on all three sides. In our practice we aim to get the applicator as close to the skin without touching as possible (▶ Fig. 6.4). It is imperative that the physician or physician extender take as much time as needed to get the applicator in close proximity to the skin. The "arm" of the device has three components that can be adjusted

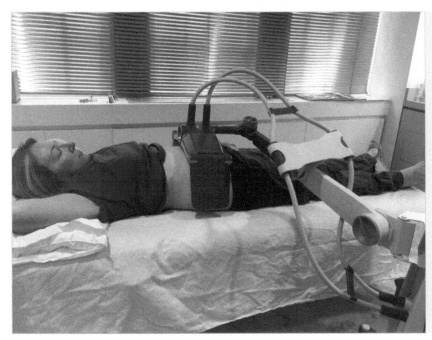

Fig. 6.3 Patient and device positioning for abdomen treatment.

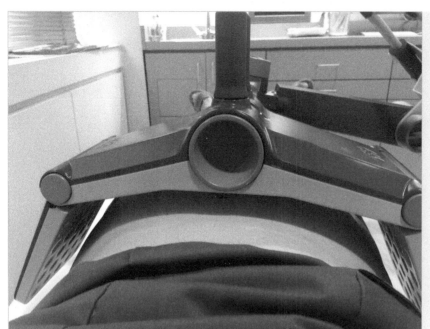

Fig. 6.4 Optimal distance from applicator to skin -10 mm.

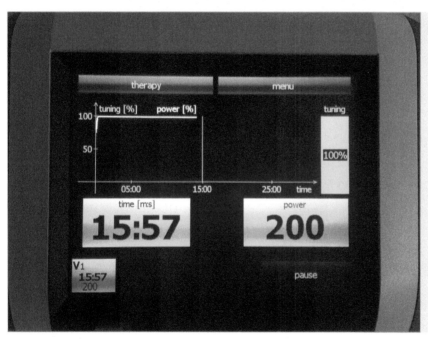

Fig. 6.5 Desired treatment setting– highest power while maintaining tuning of >90%.

independently to customize the applicator positioning to the patient's frame. The side panels are flap-like structures that can be moved up and down to further fine tune the set up. Once the set up is complete the operator can begin the treatment.

Vanquish ME offers a maximum of 200 watts of radiofrequency energy and the wattage is titrated to the highest amount possible while maintaining a tuning of greater than 90% (preferably >95%). If the tuning drops below 90%, the wattage should be decreased until it returns to a minimum of 90%, ideally 95% or greater (▶ Fig. 6.5). A common misconception is that the higher the wattage, the greater the amount of induced apoptosis that will occur, however this is not the case. Vanquish ME is most effective when operating at a wattage that provides the greatest efficiency. The output and absorption are measured and these numbers should be as close together as possible (▶ Fig. 6.6). A wide discrepancy between these two calculations indicate inefficiency, and therefore less efficacy. There are multiple reasons why the optimal wattage varies from patient to patient, and treatment to treatment in the same individual. Patients with larger amounts of subcutaneous fat will absorb more radiofrequency energy than patients with smaller treatment areas. Typically the wattage for optimal absorption decreases as patients have more treatments and the fat layer gets smaller. This may not be the case with larger patients who can sustain the highest wattage for the entire Vanquish ME series. Device operators should keep in mind that if a patient has a substantial layer of fat but is unable to maintain a high wattage throughout treatment, the applicator might be too far away from the skin. If this is the case the device can be paused to allow for repositioning of the applicator. The side panels can often be adjusted without treatment interruption. If a patient is not well-hydrated, the radiofrequency energy is unable to penetrate the skin effectively and there will be less energy available to the fat layer for absorption.

Patients and practitioners alike love the BTL Vanquish ME safety profile. Although it is technically possible for a patient to sustain a thermal injury, it is extremely unlikely when Vanquish ME treatments are set up and monitored appropriately. The Vanquish ME device is operator independent in the sense that once the device is set up there is no other manual operating required. This does not however make it a "set and forget" device. It is crucial for the safety and efficacy of the treatment for the operator to be monitoring the patient throughout the entire duration of a Vanquish ME session. The closer the device applicator is to the skin, the easier it is for the radiofrequency energy to reach the subcutaneous fat layer. This will cause more apoptosis but will also make the skin feel hotter. It is the operator's responsibility to interact with the patient to determine when the heat becomes intolerable. For most patients this will be never, but it is not uncommon to have to lift the side flap of the applicator, or turn down the wattage to give patients relief. "Hot spots" usually resolve quickly without pause in the treatment. Occasionally patients will experience a self-limiting panniculitis after Vanquish ME which feels like

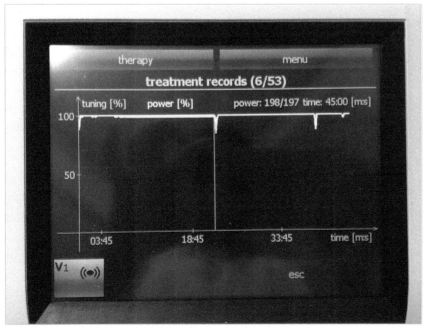

Fig. 6.6 Target output/absorption ratio is 1:1 to achieve maximum results.

a firm nodule and can be tender. Reassurance should be given that this inflammatory response surrounding a destructed fat cell will resolve once the fat cell is absorbed by the body. The metabolic process can take 2–3 weeks and it is not necessary to cease treatments during this time. Over the counter anti-inflammatory medications can be taken as needed for pain relief. Possible side effects of non-contact, selective radiofrequency treatments include mild redness and swelling for one hour or so, temporary increased skin sensitivity to heat, and occasionally, excessive sweating at the end of the treatment.[3]

Patients who are good candidates, are well-hydrated, and treated by trained practitioners can expect to see results after a series of BTL Vanquish ME (▶ Fig. 6.7). As with any surgical or non-surgical procedure results vary from person to person. A good consultation with an emphasis on realistic expectations will heavily influence a patient's perception of treatment success. A Vanquish ME series always begins with a pre-procedure set of photographs using the BTL floor mat to ensure identical foot positioning in the before and after photos. In our practice, the protocol for mid-section photographs has patients lift their arms straight out in front of them so that they are perpendicular to the body. Arms should never be lifted above shoulder height as this position stretches out the torso, distorting the baseline anatomy. In addition to photographs, it is common for providers to measure the treatment area before treatment and one month after the last treatment to quantify centimeters lost. The positioning and tension of the tape measure must be identical in the before and after measurements in order for this to be an accurate tool to assess results. The lack of reliability in circumferential measurements has led many providers to rely on photographs alone to document change. Patients see and feel the difference in their clothes and that is the ultimate gauge of success. The other methods of measuring fat reduction are caliper measurements, bioimpedance-based scale measurements, ultrasound, and most recently magnetic resonance imaging (MRI).[6]

The use of MRI is proving to be an accurate and reliable method to quantify the fat thickness reduction following Vanquish ME. A recent study published in the Journal of Drugs in Dermatology showed statistically significant results

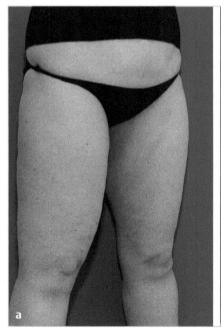
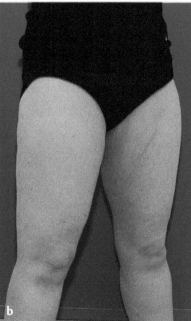

Fig. 6.7 (a, b) Before and 6 weeks after photographs of 5 Vanquish treatments to the inner/outer thighs.

in a case study that used MRI scanning to measure the difference in fat layer thickness before and after treatment. Five of the six patients enrolled in the study completed it with one patient dropping out for reasons unrelated to the study. The subjects had baseline MRI measurements of fat thickness and were measured a second time four weeks following their last Vanquish ME treatment. The abdominal area was scanned in several equidistant slices. The MRI scans were mostly obtained in dual-echo regime and exported in DICOM format for further analyses.[6] The patients completed four, 45-minute treatments, once a week for 4 weeks. The average reduction in fat layer thickness among the patients in the study was 5.36 mm. There was no significant change in patient's weight suggesting the results were in fact due to Vanquish ME rather than diet and exercise. MRI scanning is not a realistic method to measure patient results on a routine basis due to the cost of imaging, however it serves a great purpose in determining the efficacy of the technology.

BTL Vanquish ME alone will give patients circumferential fat reduction but in certain cases it is used in conjunction with other devices for synergistic effect, or as a secondary treatment. For people who have excess fat and skin laxity, a combination treatment of radiofrequency fat reduction and a skin tightening device will give patients a better result than either treatment alone. For patients who have a contour abnormality either from liposuction or cryolipolysis, Vanquish ME can often times smooth out the area of irregularity. In our experience, Vanquish ME has become a popular "gateway" procedure leading patients to other non-surgical and surgical procedures after a positive experience. We also have patients who initially opt for Vanquish ME over liposuction for the non-surgical benefits, but later go on to have liposuction to achieve even greater results. It is human nature to always want more of a good thing and once patients see a positive change in their body we find they no longer fear surgery the way they once did. For the patient who had unrealistic expectations going into a radiofrequency fat reduction series, or the rare patient who does not get a good result (less likely now that Vanquish has been upgraded to Vanquish ME), surgery might become a consideration since the non-surgical option was attempted and unsuccessful. It often times goes back to the initial consultation if a liposuction upgrade is stated as an option. A patient who feels like they were promised more than they received from radiofrequency fat reduction may look for a new practice to have surgery with. On the other hand, if a patient feels that they were well educated on the results they could expect from Vanquish ME, they are more inclined to stay "in-house" for additional procedures. We are very forthcoming with our patients regarding what they are likely to achieve with non-surgical radiofrequency fat reduction versus traditional liposuction and give a thorough consultation to all patients.

When incorporating a new non-surgical device into a practice there are many factors to consider. In addition to the device being efficacious, it has to offer a new procedure or enhance an existing one, and must make financial sense for the practice. A downside to many non-surgical devices is the cost of associated consumables. Consumable costs can be substantial and either increase procedure fees or lower the practice profit. BTL Vanquish ME does not have a consumable making it a cost-seffective device to incorporate into practice. It keeps the overhead of the device down and allows for complementary treatments if a patient would benefit from an additional session or two once a series is complete. Patients are usually appreciative of the gratis treatments and this can often times determine the overall level of satisfaction from the Vanquish ME experience.

With the success of non-contact, selective radiofrequency therapy for circumferential fat reduction came the BTL Flex applicator which is now FDA cleared to reduce fat around the thighs and saddlebags. The legs have long been a difficult area to treat non-surgically and many patients complain of unwanted fat in this area. The Flex applicator has a unique design allowing the inner and outer thigh to be treated simultaneously. The device placement can be further customized to target the upper or lower thigh depending on the patient's concerns. Treatment with the BTL Flex applicator follows the same protocol of 4–6 weekly treatments with each leg treated for 30 minutes. We have found that it takes longer than the mid-section for leg results to occur and this is likely due to the amount of fibrous connective tissue in the legs. Patients are getting results and The Aesthetic Guide reported clinical study results of 40 patients that showed an average of 1 inch reduction over four treatments of 30 minutes per leg.[7]

In the few years that we have been using selective radiofrequency for non-surgical fat reduction there have already been significant advancements in the technology. We are seeing better results with the upgraded Vanquish ME system and the Flex applicator has opened the door to treat areas outside the mid-section. Treating the legs with Vanquish ME is gaining in popularity and will only continue to do so with the new FDA clearance. Patients like the fact that they can get results without pain, anesthesia, or downtime. It will be exciting to watch the further evolution of selective radiofrequency for fat reduction. There are currently protocols being put in place to treat the upper extremities and this is likely just the beginning for this technology.

References

[1] Frentzen Jeffrey, Executive Editor, Physicians Prefer BTL Vanquish ME as Stand Alone or Adjunctive Tx, The Aesthetic Guide, 2–5, July/August 2015

[2] Weiss R, Weiss M, Beasley K, Vrba J, Bernardy J. Operator Independent Focused High Frequency ISM Band for Fat Reduction: Porcine Model Lasers Surg Med 2013; 45:235–239

[3] Fajkošová K, Machovcová A, Onder M, Fritz K. Selective radiofrequency therapy as a noninvasive approach for contactless body contouring and circumferential reduction. J Drugs Dermatol 2014; 13(3):291–296

[4] Frentzen Jeffrey, Executive Editor, Physicians Report BTL Vanquish ME Attracts Male Patients, The Aesthetic Guide, 1–4, January/February 2016

[5] Cooper JL, Salazar M. Safe, Effective Fat Reduction for Diverse Patient Populations, Supplement to Modern Aesthetics, 9–10, July/August 2015

[6] Downie J, Kaspar M. Contactless Abdominal Fat Reduction with Selective RF™ Evaluated by Magnetic Resonance Imaging (MRI): Case Study. J Drugs Dermatol 2016; 15(4):491–495

[7] Frentzen Jeffrey, Executive Editor, New BTL Flex Applicator Eases Noninvasive Thigh Treatments, The Aesthetic Guide, 2–3, January/February 2015

7 The Role of Stem Cells in Body Contouring

Aris Sterodimas

Abstract

Liposuction was designed to correct unaesthetic deposits of subcutaneous fat; it produces satisfactory silhouette contouring when performed by appropriately trained plastic surgeons using properly selected technologies. However, from lipoaspirate it is possible to obtain autologous fat graft and adipose-derived stem cells (ADSCs) for reconstructive surgery and regenerative medicine. Autologous fat transplantation uses include the correction of body contour, malformations, and post-surgical outcomes. The aim of this chapter is to highlight the crucial role of adipose tissue in plastic and reconstructive surgery, from liposuction to lipofilling and ADSCs, exposing the indications, procedures, and complications of these surgical techniques. The Stromal Enriched Lipograft (SEL) is a new surgical technique of autologous fat grafting for body contouring which converts a stem cell poor fat graft to a stem cell rich fat graft. The clinical outcomes of scientific research in the last decade have shown that SEL is one of the core elements of regenerative medicine.

Keywords: Liposuction, body contouring, lipofilling, autologous fat transplantation, adipose-derived stem cells, Stromal Enriched Lipograft

Key Points

- In this chapter, the technique, pearls, and pitfalls of SEL are described in detail. A series of patients who underwent contouring of abdomen and trunk assisted by SEL are presented.
- Careful selection of patients and proper surgical technique help avoid contour irregularity, and outcome expectations should be based on realistic preoperative evaluation of the patient's age, skin elasticity, volume of fat to be removed, and volume of fat to be transplanted.
- SEL technique aims at filling preoperatively marked deficiencies with adipocytes and adipose-derived stem cells that will survive and become incorporated into the recipient bed.
- Improvement of the gluteal contour and body contour can be attained and maintained through autologous fat transplantation by means of SEL.
- Irregularities ranging from "over suctioning" to bumpy skin and asymmetries result from an overaggressive approach to liposuction of the flanks and SEL technique can play a significant role in repairing such iatrogenic defects.

7.1 Introduction

The improvement of surgical techniques in autologous fat transplantation has increased the survival rate of the grafted fat and has reduced the side effects such as fat necrosis. Several mechanisms may contribute to the variability of outcomes for fat-grafting procedures. The harvesting process is traumatic to adipocytes, which can lead to apoptosis. Additionally, results for recipient wound beds with different degrees of blood supply and fluctuations in oxygen delivery may range from adequate revascularization and good "take" to insufficient revascularization and ischemia, apoptosis, and dedifferentiation of central adipocytes.[1] A significant proportion of the engrafted fat undergoes resorption and necrosis due to the non-vascularized nature of the transplant. Resorption rates after fat grafting are generally reported to be between 20 and 80%.[2] Therefore, in order to maximize survival, multiple passes in different tissue planes are required in order to optimize plasmatic imbibition and neo-vascularization of the transplanted fat grafts. Injection of the fat graft should be met with minimal resistance and a small volume is administered upon entry with the remaining volume given during withdrawal to minimize trauma. Adipose tissue is composed of mature adipocytes constituting about 90% of the tissue volume, and a stromal vascular fraction (SVF) including fibroblasts, endothelial cells, preadipocytes, vascular smooth muscle cells, lymphocytes, resident monocytes/macrophages. It has become apparent over the years that white adipose tissue (WAT) is the most suitable autologous injectable filler for correcting soft tissue defects.[3] Adipose tissue is considered as a source of mesenchymal stem cells (MSCs), termed adipose-derived stem cells (ADSCs). They are ubiquitous and easily obtained in large quantities with little donor site morbidity or patient discomfort making the use of autologous ADSCs an appropriate cellular therapy. The use of ASCs may enhance angiogenesis, improve the survival of grafts, and thus reduce atrophy of the fat grafting.[4] ADSCs have been evaluated in clinical studies for soft tissue augmentation and represent a novel approach to cell-based therapies, such as autologous fat transplantation. Nowadays, autologous fat transplantation or adipose cell grafting incorporates adipocytes, ADSCs and growth factors already present in the lipoaspirate. The SEL is a new surgical technique of autologous fat grafting for body contouring which converts a stem cell poor fat graft to a stem cell rich fat graft.[5] The clinical outcomes of scientific research in the last decade have shown that SEL is one of the core elements of regenerative medicine.

7.2 Patient Selection

Body contouring of the trunk and extremities combines liposuction, excisional surgical techniques, and autologous fat grafting.[6] Body contouring patients should be carefully evaluated for their expectations and the actual results that can be achieved by this procedure. Planning the procedure and indicating it properly is just as important as the surgical procedure itself. Patients who clearly have any psychiatric disorder, such as body dysmorphic disorder are referred for psychiatric evaluation. However there are subtle cases in which patients present low self-esteem, borderline type of anxiety, and unrealistic expectations. In those cases, sometimes it is better to deny operating on the patient. The ideal patient for body contouring procedures has a small amount of adipose tissue to be suctioned out in order to improve the body contour, has small skin laxity, and is dedicated to a healthy lifestyle, including daily physical exercise and a healthy diet. It is the responsibility of the surgeon to address all concerns, risks, goals and expectations of the procedure chosen for the patient in order to avoid false expectations and future frustrations. In this chapter we will address special attention to trunk and thighs including the following areas: upper and lower abdomen, upper and lower back, flanks, pubis and sacrum V-zone, gluteal area, inner thighs, outer thighs, inner knees, and banana rolls.

7.3 Technique

Marking of the areas to be liposuctioned are made while the patient is in standing position. Preoperative sedation in the surgical suite is administered.

Anesthesia consists of an epidural block and intravenous sedation. The patient is placed in prone position. After the injection of normal saline wetting solution containing 1:500,000 of adrenaline by a small-bore cannula and waiting 15 minutes, a 60-cc syringe attached to a 4 mm blunt cannula is inserted through small incisions. Fat is aspirated by using the syringe method. The 2/3 of the aspirated fat is used in order to isolate the SVF. Digestion is done with 0.075% collagenase (Sigma, St. Louis, MO) in buffered saline and agitated for 30 minutes at 37°C in Celltibator (Medikan, Los Angeles, CA). Separation of the SVF containing ADSCs is then done by using centrifugation at 1200 × g for 5 minutes. The Lipokit Centrifuge (Medikan, Los Angeles, CA), is used. The SVF is located in the pellet derived from the centrifuged fat at the bottom of the lipoaspirate. In SEL, freshly isolated SVF is attached to the aspirated fat, with the fat tissue acting as a living bioscaffold before transplantation.[7] The remaining 1/3 of the aspirated fat is treated in the following manner: with the syringe held vertically with the open end down, the fat and fluid are separated. Isotonic saline is added to the syringe, the fat and saline are separated and the exudate discarded. The procedure is repeated until the fat becomes yellow in color, free of blood and other contaminants.[8] Mixing of the SVF containing ADSCs and the purified fat is then done (▶ Fig. 7.1). This whole procedure is done inside the operating theatre, by 2 tissue engineers, manually, and the time required is about 90 minutes. Tissue planes are created by using specific cannulas in different trajectories, always from the deeper aspect to more

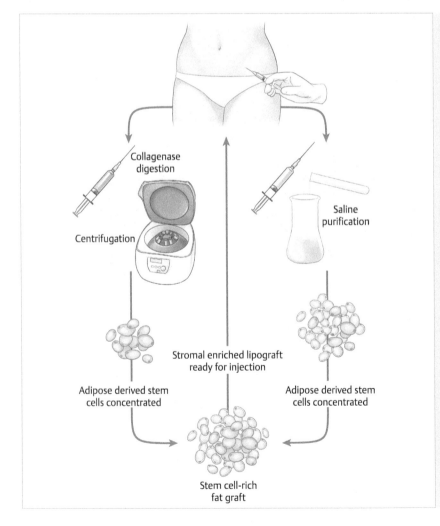

Fig. 7.1 Schematic representation of Stromal Enriched Lipograft technique.

Collagenase digestion

Centrifugation

Saline purification

Adipose derived stem cells concentrated

Stromal enriched lipograft ready for injection

Adipose derived stem cells concentrated

Stem cell-rich fat graft

superficial areas. Successful fat application is performed using a blunt cannula that creates a tunnel at insertion and the fat is injected as the cannula is withdrawn in order to avoid intravascular fat injection. Multiple passes are used to fan across the deficient region. Antibiotics, analgesics, and anti-inflammatory medications are prescribed during the following 7 postoperative days.

7.4 Clinical Applications

SEL technique aims at filling preoperatively marked deficiencies with adipocytes that will survive and become incorporated into the recipient bed. The combination of circumferential liposuction, SEL of buttocks and lower limbs in a single surgical procedure has been performed successfully in the last 10 years, emphasizing the low rate of complications and the high overall patient satisfaction.[9] SEL should be thought as part of body contouring in order to give the balanced and properly proportioned anatomy of the body. The aspirated fat may be utilized to augment, shape, and to correct irregularities or asymmetry that may be detected preoperatively.[10] The use of SEL for body contouring has gained attention due to further improvements in the fat preparation and processing. Recently the concept of composite body contouring has been introduced where combining lipoabdominoplasty and SEL to the thighs and gluteal area has been done in 375 patients with aesthetically favorable results.

7.4.1 Patient 1

This 34-year-old lady presented complaining of gluteal contour depression after suffering a trauma in her left buttock area which made her "unattractive". Preoperative views of the patient are shown (▶Fig. 7.2). Liposuction of the back, flanks, and abdomen and SEL was performed in the left gluteal area. The total gluteal fat transfer was 350 mL. Postoperative views taken 3 years after the procedure (▶Fig. 7.3).

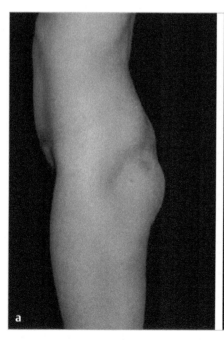
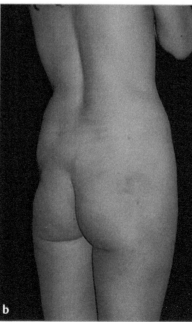

Fig. 7.2 (a, b) Preoperative views of a 34-year-old lady presented complaining of gluteal contour depression after suffering a trauma in her left buttock area.

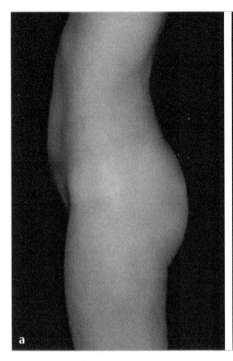
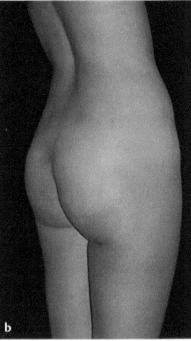

Fig. 7.3 (a, b) Postoperative views of a 34-year-old lady 3 years after SEL was performed in the left gluteal area. The total gluteal fat transfer was 350 mL.

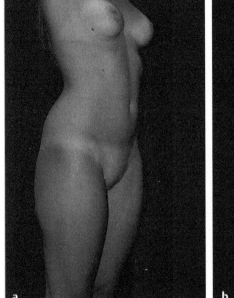
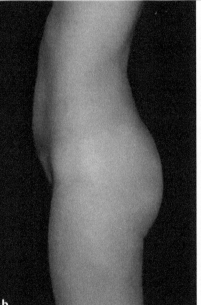
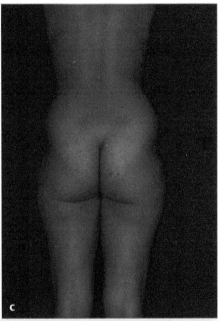

Fig. 7.4 (a–c) Preoperative views of a 28-year-old woman presented for liposuction and moderate buttock enhancement.

7.4.2 Patient 2

This 28-year-old woman presented for liposuction and moderate buttock enhancement. Preoperative views of the patient are shown (▶ Fig. 7.4). Liposuction of the back, flanks, and abdomen was done. SEL was performed. The total gluteal fat transfer was 350 mL per side. Postoperative views taken 4 years after the procedure (▶ Fig. 7.5).

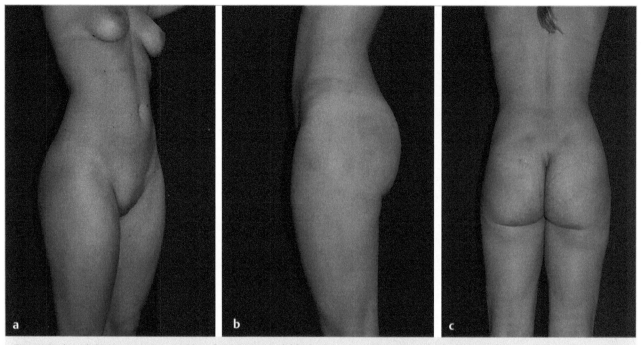

Fig. 7.5 (a–c) Postoperative views of a 34-year-old lady 4 years after SEL was performed in the gluteal area per side. The total gluteal fat transfer was 350 mL.

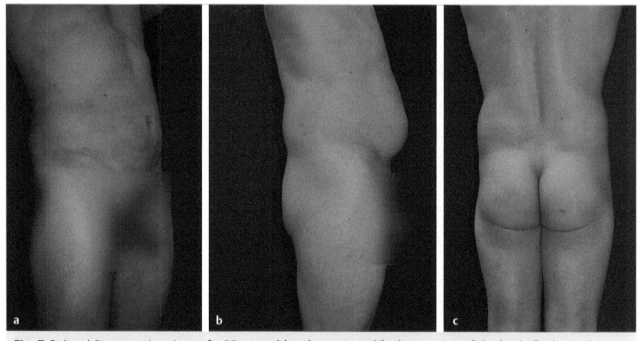

Fig. 7.6 (a–c) Preoperative views of a 35-year-old male presented for liposuction of the back, flanks, and abdomen and SEL was performed.

7.4.3 Patient 3

This 35-year-old man complained about his body shape. Preoperative views of the patient are shown (▶ Fig. 7.6). Liposuction of the back, flanks, and abdomen and SEL was performed. The total gluteal fat transfer was 170 mL per side using the SEL technique. Postoperative views taken 2 years after the procedure (▶ Fig. 7.7).

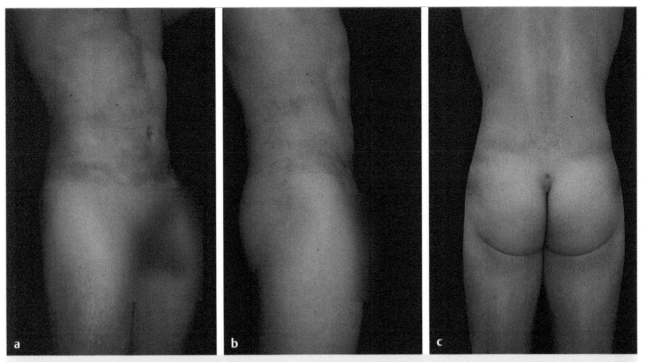

Fig. 7.7 (a–c) Postoperative views of a 35-year-old male 2 years after SEL was performed in the gluteal area per side. The total gluteal fat transfer was 170 mL.

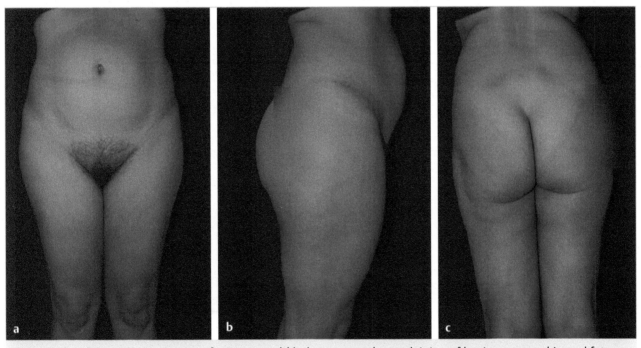

Fig. 7.8 (a–c) Preoperative views of a 51-year-old lady presented complaining of having excess skin and fat deposits which made her "unattractive".

7.4.4 Patient 4

This 51-year-old lady presented complaining of having excess skin and fat deposits which made her "unattractive". Preoperative views are shown (▶Fig. 7.8). Liposuction of the back, flanks, lipoabdominoplasty and SEL was performed. The total gluteal fat transfer was 520 mL per side using the SEL technique. Postoperative views taken 4 years after the procedure (▶Fig. 7.9).

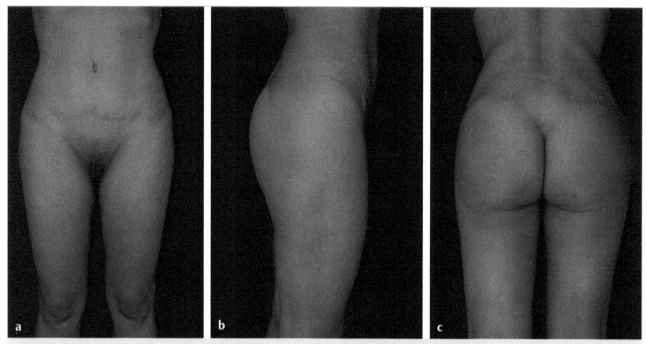

Fig. 7.9 (a–c) Postoperative views of a 51-year-old lady 4 years after undergoing liposuction of the back, flanks, lipoabdominoplasty and SEL in the gluteal area. The total gluteal fat transfer was 520 mL per side using the SEL technique.

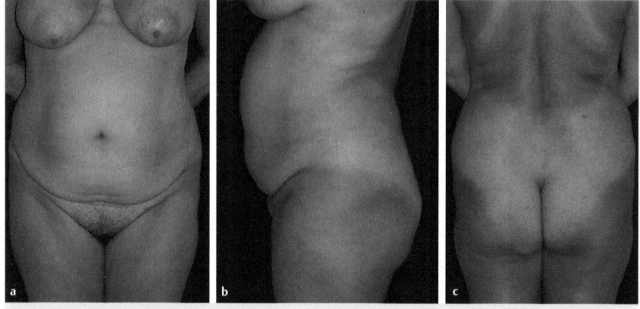

Fig. 7.10 (a–c) Preoperative views of a 73-year-old lady presented complaining of having excess skin and fat deposits which made her "unattractive".

7.4.5 Patient 5

This 73-year-old woman presented complaining of having excess skin and fat deposits which made her "unattractive". Preoperative views are shown (▶Fig. 7.10). Liposuction of the back, flanks, lipoabdominoplasty and SEL was performed. The total gluteal fat transfer was 620 mL per

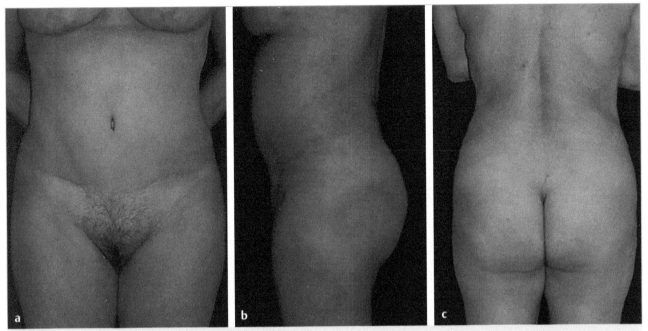

Fig. 7.11 (a–c) Postoperative views of a 73-year-old lady 2 years after undergoing liposuction of the back, flanks, lipoabdominoplasty and SEL in the gluteal area. The total gluteal fat transfer was 620 mL per side using the SEL technique.

side using the SEL technique. Postoperative views taken 2 years after the procedure (▶Fig. 7.11).

7.5 Discussion

Fat grafting for body contouring remains shrouded in the stigma of variable results experienced by most plastic surgeons when they first graft fat. The need for standardization of autologous fat grafting technique needs to be done. Numerous clinical reports have been published regarding techniques of fat graft harvesting, preparation, and injection. Techniques are still selected according to a surgeon's individual preference, since quantitative evidence of clinical fat survivability and predictability of volume restoration does not exist. ADSCs can be distinguished from other adipocyte progenitor populations based on their expression of a variety of surface markers. The regenerative capacity of ADSCs during graft setting and their contribution to fat regeneration remains undefined. Clinical studies have demonstrated that the resident ADSCs within fat grafted tissues can differentiate into adipocytes and add structure to fill the implanted tissue defect; secrete growth factors, cytokines, and chemo-attractants that can enhance angiogenesis and increase local vascularization and blood supply; and inhibit innate immune responses after tissue transplantation.[11] Recent studies have indicated that ADSCs can promote angiogenesis in addition to suppressing inflammation. An accepted principle of autologous fat grafting is that adipocytes survive only when within 2 mm of an arterial blood supply. Fat cells outside this boundary may undergo necrosis leading to scar tissue. The adipose tissue graft enriched with SVF is woven into the targeted tissues, injecting only 5–10 mL of fat with each pass as in order to obtain the most reliable clinical outcome. The process of fat regeneration is progressed by ADSCs between 3 and 7 days, so the role of

ASC is important in fat grafting. ADSCs are also involved with establishing fat homeostasis. These properties support successful tissue regeneration and the long-term survival of the fat graft. It has been shown that ADSCs harvested from superficial abdominal regions are significantly more resistant to apoptosis than other parts.[12]

Recent clinical series show that adipose-derived stem cells offer the possibility of finally fulfilling the key principle of replacing like with like as an aesthetic filler, without the drawbacks of current technology. In SEL, autologous adipose-derived stem cells (ADSCs) are used in combination with lipoinjection. A stromal vascular fraction (SVF) containing ADSCs is freshly isolated from half of the aspirated fat and recombined with the other half. This process converts relatively ADSC-poor aspirated fat to ADSC-rich fat. SEL is based on the use of adipose-derived stem cells combined with a biomaterial that is the adipose tissue that has been processed to be used as a natural scaffold and biomolecules, cytokines, and growth factors, which are secreted by the stem cells and the adipose tissue. A recents study has confirmed that the SEL fat can survive better than non-SEL fat, and microvasculature can be detected more prominently in SEL fat, especially in the outer layers of the fat transfer.[13]

References

[1] Sterodimas A, Boriani F, Magarakis E, Nicaretta B, Pereira LH, Illouz YG. Thirty four years of liposuction: past, present and future. Eur Rev Med Pharmacol Sci 2012;16(3):393–406

[2] Sterodimas A, De Faria J, Correa WE, Pitanguy I. Tissue engineering in plastic surgery: an up-to-date review of the current literature. Ann Plast Surg 2009;62(1):97–103

[3] Sterodimas A, de Faria J, Nicaretta B, Pitanguy I. Tissue engineering with adipose-derived stem cells (ADSCs): current and future applications. J Plast Reconstr Aesthet Surg 2010;63(11):1886–1892

[4] Sterodimas A, de Faria J, Nicaretta B, Papadopoulos O, Papalambros E, Illouz YG. Cell-assisted lipotransfer. Aesthet Surg J 2010;30(1):78–81

[5] Sterodimas A, Illouz YG. Conclusions and future directions In: Adipose derived stem cells and regenerative medicine. Eds Illouz YG, Sterodimas A. Springer-Verlag Berlin Heidelberg 2011:273–276

[6] Pereira LH, Sterodimas A. Composite body contouring. Aesthetic Plast Surg 2009;33(4):616–624

[7] Sterodimas A. Stromal enriched lipograft for rhinoplasty refinement. Aesthet Surg J 2013;33(4):612–614

[8] Sterodimas A, Huanquipaco JC, de Souza Filho S, Bornia FA, Pitanguy I. Autologous fat transplantation for the treatment of Parry-Romberg syndrome. J Plast Reconstr Aesthet Surg 2009;62(11):e424–e426

[9] Sterodimas A, de Faria J, Nicaretta B, Boriani F. Autologous fat transplantation versus adipose-derived stem cell-enriched lipografts: a study. Aesthet Surg J 2011;31(6):682–693

[10] Nicareta B, Pereira LH, Sterodimas A, Illouz YG. Autologous gluteal lipograft. Aesthetic Plast Surg 2011;35(2):216–224

[11] Sterodimas A, Pereira LH. Liposuction of the abdomen and trunk In: Rubin JP, Jewell ML, Richter D, eds. Body Contouring & liposuction. New York, NY: Uebel CO W.B. Saunders Elsevier; 2012:311–320

[12] Sterodimas A. Adipose Stem Cell Engineering: Clinical applications in plastic and reconstructive surgery In: Illouz YG, Sterodimas A, eds. Adipose derived stem cells and regenerative medicine. Berlin Heidelberg: Springer-Verlag; 2011:165–180

[13] Sterodimas A. Tissue Engineering with adipose-derived stem cells (ADSCs) in plastic and reconstructive surgery: current and future applications In: Di Giussepe A, Shiffman M, eds. New Frontiers in plastic and cosmetic surgery. PA, USA: The Health Sciences Publisher; 2015:3–11

8 Ethnic Considerations in Liposuction

William Lao

Abstract

Liposuction is an individualized procedure. With the increasing globalization, plastic surgeons are constantly faced with patients from different backgrounds. This chapter discusses the differences in ideal body type, body mass index, skin makeup, and scar tendency in different ethnic groups.

Keywords: Liposuction, ethnic ideals, body shaping, liposuction scar, liposculpture

8.1 Introduction

The practice environment for plastic surgeons nowadays has changed tremendously both internationally and domestically. Internet has substantially modified our way of living and shrunk the world we live in. To plastic surgeons, the social network and various Internet platforms are now essential components of practice advertisement and patient recruitment strategies. These platforms have also provided more opportunities for international consultations and their eventual procedures. Domestically, the population make up of each nation is more diversified than ever. The United States, for example, has seen a tremendous growth of the minority population. From 2000 to 2010, there is a percentage drop of the Caucasian population from 75 to 63% while experiencing a concomitant growth of the Hispanic and Asian population from 12.5 to 16.3% and 3.6 to 4.7%, respectively.[1] Further it is estimated that by 2050, Hispanic will become the largest minority and comprise of 24% of the nation's population.[2]

As the population structure changes, so is the make up of our cosmetic patients. Cosmetic patients in the USA have predominately been Caucasian in the past; however, in the last decade, there has been a steady growth of cosmetic surgery performed in ethnic minorities. A 10-year retrospective analysis showed from 1998 to 2007, there were actually 1.8% decline in Caucasian cosmetic patients but increases of 7.5%, 4.7%, 14.5%, and 105.5% in Black, Hispanic, Asian, and native American patients, respectively.[3] More recent data from the ASPS in 2015, Asian Americans represent 7% of all cosmetic procedures; Black and Hispanic represent 9% and 11%, respectively (▶Table 8.1). All minority groups combined to 31% of all cosmetic procedures performed in 2015 and continued to have positive growth from 2014.[4]

One thing that remains constant is the popularity of liposuction procedure. Across ethnic groups, liposuction continues to be one of the top cosmetic procedures performed.[2] Since each culture has its own preferences and cosmetic ideals, as a plastic surgeon of the 21st century, it is of paramount importance to understand the different needs of patients from various ethnic backgrounds.

Table 8.1 2015 cosmetic demographics in the United States

Ethnicity breakdown of cosmetic procedures	2015	% 2015	2014	% 2014	% change 2015 vs. 2014
Caucasian	10,969,059	69%	10,819,104	69%	1%
Hispanic	1,688,714	11%	1,633,598	10%	3%
African–American	1,362,282	9%	1,324,779	8%	3%
Asian–American	1,093,720	7%	1,078,497	7%	1%
Other	794,555	5%	766,888	5%	4%

Approximately 1/3 of all cosmetic procedures in 2015 were done in ethnic minorities.
Source: 2015 Plastic Surgery Statistics Report. ASPS http://www.plasticsurgery.org/Documents/news-resources/statistics/2015-statistics/cosmetic-procedures-ethnicity.pdf Accessed September 1st, 2016.

8.2 Ideal Body Shape

To define the ideal body shape for any culture or even a small group of people is an impossible task. "Beauty is in the eye of the beholder", and how the beholder identifies beauty often comes from his/her own cultural upbringing and fashion trends of the time. Throughout history we see examples of cultural beauty like the foot binding in ancient China, elongated neck with brass coils in the Kayan tribe, and the corset binding of the Victorian era. These now seemingly extreme standards of beauty were once considered norm in the societies then.

With the current globalization, however, standard of beauty and fashion for the first time unifies and influences the world instantly a few mouse clicks away. The less common ideals of beauty mentioned above are not seen and most beauty magazines around the world portrait images of beautiful men or women with more or less variations of a theme.

We as plastic surgeons also have tried to standardize beauty with measured proportions and defined beauty from ideal population norms like the Penn numbers for breast and nipple measurements and Gunter's nasal measurements.[5,6] Liposuction, compared to rhinoplasty, has less variation of the ideal goal across cultures.

For liposuction of the arms and legs, the goal is always to restore the youthful, tightened cylindrical shape if the skin elasticity is appropriate. As for the trunk, an hour-glassed curve from the breast to waist then hip is desired across all ethnicities (▶Fig. 8.1). Singh et al further defined 0.7 as the ideal waist to hip circumference ratio across culture.[7] Though this ratio can be followed as the general guideline, there are variations of the shape preference in the buttock region; paying attention to these details will reward you with higher patient satisfaction. The list below identifies the general ethnic buttock ideals in the USA (▶Fig. 8.2).

• African American: Though 0.7 is cited in many studies as the ideal waist to hip ratio, smaller waist to hip ratio (WHR) is often tolerated and desired. A study showed that African American men are more likely to choose a lower WHR as ideal compared to their Caucasian counterpart.[8] This means a more exaggerated curve between the waist and hip. Very full lateral buttock and lateral thighs are often desired; liposuction of these areas is to be avoided.

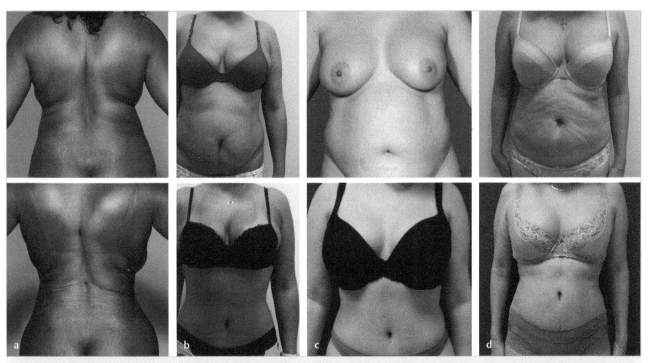

Fig. 8.1 (a–d) Hour-glass shaped trunk is desired across cultures. In order: Pre- and postoperative photos of satisfied African American, Hispanic, Caucasian, and Asian patients after liposuction with/without abdominoplasty to accentuate the hour-glassed shape in the trunk.

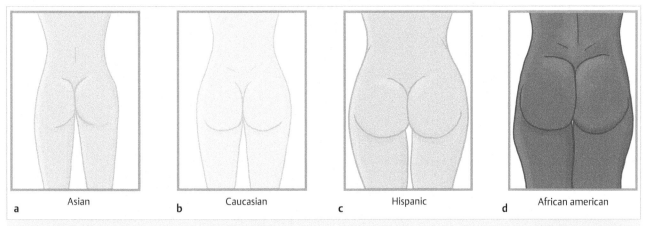

Fig. 8.2 (a–d) Graphic representation of buttock ideals among different ethnic groups in the USA. Asian: Small, shaped buttock with no lateral buttock and lateral thigh fullness; Caucasian: Moderate size buttock with lateral buttock fullness but no lateral thigh fullness; Hispanic: Full buttock with lateral buttock fullness and moderate lateral thigh fullness; African American: Full buttock with a "shelf" superiorly with lateral buttock fullness and lateral thigh fullness at the junction of buttock and thigh.

Often times they might actually request these areas to be fat grafted. While a gentle posterior inward curve from the buttock to lower back is favored in all ethnic groups, African Americans often prefer an exaggerated lordosis with a shelf formed by the superior buttock. Also for many African Americans, the lateral trochanter area is considered the hip, instead of the common iliac crest area.[9]

- Hispanic: A very full lateral buttocks is also preferred but only slight fullness of the lateral thigh is desired compared to African Americans.[9]
- Caucasian: Either a rounded lateral buttock or a hollow athletic shape is preferred.[9] No lateral thigh fullness is desired, so this area along with the medial thighs are often requested to be shaped with liposuction.
- Asian: No lateral thigh or lateral buttock fullness is preferred. These areas are often requested to be liposuctioned by Asian patients. Asian pelvis is usually smaller than other ethnic groups so less liposuction volume can achieve the same or greater effects.[10] Asian patients also tend to use liposuction for shaping rather than for total body fat reduction. The BMI in Asian patients is typically normal already, they often come in for a specific part of their body where fat tends to accumulate, ie. medial or lateral thighs, love handles, and posterior flanks. There are, but less common, full body liposuction requested compared to the other groups.

These descriptions are generalizations of the ethnic patients specifically in the United States. There are of course individual variations within a certain ethnic group. The environmental influence is also great. There are studies that showed African Americans picking up more Caucasian ideals of beauty when they moved into the Caucasian social circle, and vice versa.[11] Differences between nations also apply. While thinness is valued equally high in a study comparing the body perceptions of American students and Chinese students, the students in China value slenderness with plumpness while American students value slenderness with an athletic and firm muscular look.[12]

8.3 BMI Differences

Obesity is pandemic especially in the United States. Over 1/3 of the US population is obese in 2012.[13] There are also significant differences if we look into the ethnic subgroups (▶ Table 8.2). Obesity is most prevalent in the African American and Hispanic groups, estimated 47.8% and 42.5% of the subgroup populations have a BMI >30, respectively.[13]

The prevalence of obesity in African Americans could be partly explained by their greater tolerance to larger body shapes and BMI. Coetzee et al showed that the African American ideal BMI is heavier than the Caucasian ideal BMI.[14] Another study of Caucasian and African American college students also showed that African American men are more likely to pick model figures heavier than their Caucasian counterparts.[8] These preferences partly explain why

Table 8.2 Prevalence of obesity in different ethnic groups in the United States in 2012

	Asian	Caucasian	Hispanic	African American
% Population BMI >30	10.8%	32.6%	42.5%	47.8%

Source: Adapted from Ogden CL, Carroll MD, Kit BK, Flegal KM. Prevalence of obesity among adults: United States, 2011–2012. NCHS Data Brief. No. 131, October 2013.

heavier weight is more prevalent in the African American population aside from other socioeconomics issues.

Asian American only consists of a small percentage of the obesity population; only 10% in the USA are considered obese.[13] The intrinsic differences in BMI and obesity help to explain why Asian patients request liposuction more for shaping than fat reduction compared to the other ethnic groups.

Due to the lower BMI, Asians typically have a more slender built. Often times, this is the more desired body form from the Western ideal of curvy body shape in young girls. For surgeons who are not familiar with this slender Asian ideal, they might think the already thin Asian patient requesting liposuction has body dysmorphic syndrome. While it's pertinent to screen for that, it is also important to understand the Asian mentality for the pursuit of ultra-thinness. A study done on female college students in Taiwan with an average BMI of 20 mostly preferred study figures thinner than their perception of current figure, the figure as others saw them, and the figure they felt most of the time.[15] Plastic surgeons in other parts of the world have to understand this constant pursuit to be thinner in Asians.

8.4 Skin Quality

There are intrinsic differences between the skin make up and aging process of the different ethnic groups. One study showed that the African American skin retains more of its elasticity and thickness compared to its Caucasian counterpart. Specifically, the dermal-epidermal junction flattens and thins with aging and this process occurs in a lesser and slower degree in African American compared to Caucasian.[16] Asian also has a thicker dermis than Caucasian.[17] These facts might contribute to the more youthful looking skin in African Americans and Asians compared to Caucasians of the same age. There are also genetic and environmental factors that influence the aging of skin. Caucasian skin compared to Asian and African American skin already produces less amount of the sun protective melanin yet Caucasian cultures enjoy activities like sun tanning more than other ethnic groups. The previous study also showed a decrease dermal-epidermal junction thickness in sun-exposed areas.[16] So the author firmly believes that the genetically more vulnerable skin plus sun tanning habit act together as double threats to the more pronounced skin aging in Caucasians. This can partly explain why facelift is more often done in the Caucasian population, less so in Asian, and even more rare in the African American population at the same age.

The same skin changes apply to body skin as well. Caucasian skin is less elastic and more likely to require skin excision surgeries like the abdominoplasty, thighlift, and brachioplasty in addition to liposuction to restore a youthful form. Whereas in Asian and African Americans, because of the better skin elasticity in general, it is more feasible to perform liposuction first and if needed staged the skin excision later.

8.5 Attitude toward General Anesthesia

Having practiced both in the United States and Asia, I noticed an unknown fear for general anesthesia in Asia. Personally, general anesthesia with a protected airway is safer than IV sedation. Many Asian patients, however, have an unknown fear for general anesthesia and they would rather tolerate a small amount of pain and discomfort and elect to undergo surgery with just local anesthesia or IV sedation. When I practiced in Asia, I had to adapt doing most procedures like lower blepharoplasty and even facial fat grafting with harvest all under local anesthesia. This seemingly common modality for Asian plastic surgeons might not be so familiar for surgeons from the United States.

It is also popular to do liposuction for a specific area under local anesthesia. Generally 2000 to 3000 cc of liposuction can be well tolerated with patient completely awake using only tumescent solution.

8.6 Scarring

Plastic surgeons always make an effort to hide the liposuction scar in creases or intersection of two surfaces. The idea of asymmetrical placement of the liposuction entrance wounds when doing bilateral procedures should be practiced to avoid the telltale scars of liposuction. In most Caucasian patients, the liposuction scars mature well with thin hypopigmentation. With the light skin color, these scars are barely visible. In certain ethnic groups like the Asian and African American, hyperpigmentation of the scar is more likely. Paying attention to the scar placement is even more important also because of the higher probability of hypertrophic scar and keloid formation.[18] Incisions should be avoided in the keloid prone areas like the anterior chest, neck, scapular region, suprapubic region, and joints.[19] Fewer entrance sites are preferred and better utilization of each site to maximize regional liposuction should be considered.

Although both Asian and African Americans are more prone to keloid and hypertrophic scar than Caucasians, the author believes that Asian patients tend to show their scar more than African Americans due to the stronger color contrast (▶ Fig. 8.3). Many Asians have relatively pale skin and once unsightly scars form, they often are even more obvious than the same color scar on an African American patient. Therefore, thorough communication before surgery and careful scar management after surgery are paramount in these darker skinned ethnic patients.

Mentally, Asians are also less tolerant to scars than other ethnic groups. The idea of having any type of scar has come up as a frequent reason for denying surgeries. This is another reason why non-surgical devices are more popular in Asia.

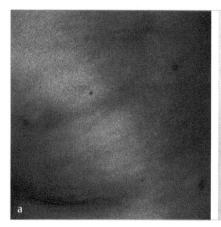 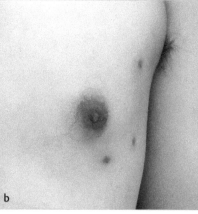

Fig. 8.3 Hyperpigmentation in African American and Asian liposuction entrance wounds. Similar scar hyperpigmentation at 4 months after surgery can appear more obvious in paler Asian patients due to the color contrast. On the left (**a**), liposuction scar near buttock area in an African American female. On the right (**b**), liposuction scars near the lateral chest in an Asian male.

Plastic surgeons should also pay attention to the clothing a specific culture tends to wear. In an interesting paper on liposuction scars in different cultures, an Indian surgeon points out the need to avoid scars in the central abdomen because this area is often exposed when Indian women wear their traditional cloth, Saree. The entrance sites for gynecomastia liposuction in Indian men should be carefully selected as well because they are often bare-chested during prayers.[20] It should be routine to show the patient preoperatively where the scars are planned.

8.7 Conclusion

Liposuction is always an individualized procedure. There are, however, general ideal body types requested by each ethnic group. In this day and age, plastic surgeons have a more diverse population to serve and should be familiar with the minor differences in body shaping, healing tendencies, and also the mentalities of different ethnic groups. A surgeon having this unique set of knowledge not only appears more professional and considerate to the patient during a consultation, but also leads to potentially higher postoperative satisfaction.

References

[1] U.S. Census Bureau. National Population Estimates: Decennial Census. Available at: https://www.census.gov/popest/data/. Accessed September 1, 2016

[2] Wimalawansa S. McKnight Aisha, Bullocks JM. Socioeconomic impact of ethnic cosmetic surgery: trends and potential financial impact the African American, Asian American, Latin American, and Middle Eastern have on cosmetic surgery. Semin Plast Surg 2009; 23(3):159–162

[3] Prendergast TI, Ong'uti SK, Ortega G, et al. Differential trends in racial preferences for cosmetic surgery procedures. Am Surg 2011; 77(8):1081–1085

[4] American Society of Plastic Surgeons. 2015 Cosmetic Demographics. Available at: http://www.plasticsurgery.org/Documents/news-resources/statistics/2015-statistics/cosmetic-procedures-ethnicity.pdf. Accessed September 1, 2016

[5] Penn J. Breast reduction. Br J Plast Surg 1955; 7(4):357–371

[6] Gunter JP. Facial analysis for the rhinoplasty patient. Dallas Rhinoplasty Symp 1993; 10:1728

[7] Singh D. Adaptive significance of female physical attractiveness: role of waist-to-hip ratio. J Pers Soc Psychol 1993; 65(2):293–307

[8] Freedman REK, Carter MM, Sbrocco T, Gray JJ. Ethnic differences in preferences for female weight and waist-to-hip ratio: a comparison of African-American and White American college and community samples. Eat Behav 2004; 5(3):191–198

[9] Roberts TL, III, Weinfeld AB, Bruner TW, Nguyen K. "Universal" and ethnic ideals of beautiful buttocks are best obtained by autologous micro fat grafting and liposuction. Clin Plast Surg 2006; 33(3):371–394

[10] Park TH, Whang KW. Buttock reshaping with intramuscular gluteal augmentation in an Asian ethnic group. Ann Plast Surg 2014; 00(00):1–8

[11] Lee EI, Roberts TL, Bruner TW. Ethnic considerations in buttock aesthetics. Semin Plast Surg 2009; 23(3):232–243

[12] Chen W, Swalm RL. Chinese and American college students' body-image: perceived body shape and body affect. Percept Mot Skills 1998; 87(2):395–403

[13] Ogden CL, Carroll MD, Kit BK, Flegal KM. Prevalence of obesity among adults: United States, 20112012. NCHS Data Brief 2013(131):1–8

[14] Coetzee V, Perrett DI. African and Caucasian body ideals in South Africa and the United States. Eat Behav 2011; 12(1):72–74

[15] Shih MY, Kubo C. Body shape preference and body satisfaction in Taiwanese college students. Psychiatry Res 2002; 111(23):215–228

[16] Querleux B, Baldeweck T, Diridollou S, et al. Skin from various ethnic origins and aging: an in vivo cross-sectional multimodality imaging study. Skin Res Technol 2009; 15(3):306–313

[17] Kim S, Choi TH, Liu W, Ogawa R, Suh JS, Mustoe TA. Update on scar management: guidelines for treating Asian patients. Plast Reconstr Surg 2013; 132(6):1580–1589

[18] Alhady SM, Sivanantharajah K. Keloids in various races. A review of 175 cases. Plast Reconstr Surg 1969; 44(6):564–566

[19] Ogawa R. Scar management for Asian cosmetic surgery patients. In: Pu LLQ, eds. Aesthetic Plastic Surgery in Asians

[20] Field LM. Cultural and ethnic differences in the acceptance or rejection of liposuction instrumentation entrance marks. J Drugs Dermatol 2007; 6(1):56–58

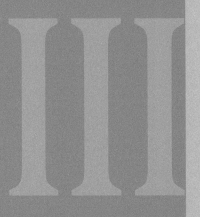

Section III

Liposuction Technology

9 Laser-Assisted Liposuction Under Local Anesthesia: Office-Based Surgery

Christopher T. Chia

Abstract

Suction-assisted lipectomy (SAL) remains one of the top cosmetic procedures worldwide. The overwhelming majority of cases are performed under general anesthesia or with intravenous sedation. With the addition of energy-assisted liposuction modalities such as laser, ultrasound, radiofrequency and power-assist, body contouring outcomes become more predictable and reproducible. Combining these with the technique of local anesthesia in an office-based surgical facility has many advantages including avoidance of general anesthesia, faster recuperative time, an excellent safety profile, and lower cost to both the patient and practitioner alike. For the body contouring aesthetic surgeon, the cornerstone of effective SAL under local anesthesia (with and without energy-assisting modalities) is the complete understanding of proper lidocaine dosing, its effective administration, its metabolism by the body as well as the risks for toxicity. The goal of this chapter is to introduce the concepts and techniques of safe and effective energy-assisted liposuction in an office-based surgery setting.

Keywords: Tumescent anesthesia, local anesthesia, lidocaine, suction-assisted lipectomy, liposuction, body contouring safety

9.1 Introduction

Irrespective of whether the surgeon decides to incorporate energy of any kind with their SAL body contouring cases, an extensive understanding of fluid dynamics, anesthesia parameters, and an improved concept of appropriate indications is critical for safety and superior aesthetic outcomes. All SAL cases involve injection of varying amounts of an isotonic solution together with dilute lidocaine and epinephrine into the subcutaneous adipose layer, resulting in analgesia both intra-operatively and postoperatively. Vasoconstriction due to the epinephrine effect minimizes blood loss. The use of the tumescent technique in liposuction has been proven to be safe with a very low morbidity and mortality rate. Worldwide, the overwhelming majority of cases are performed under general anesthesia which has many advantages but may carry a small but significant risk to the patient. More recently, performing SAL has increased in number due to the advantages of avoidance of general anesthesia, faster recuperative time, excellent safety profile and lower cost.

Over the past two decades, various methods of delivering energy into the subcutaneous fat space have been developed. These include ultrasonic-assisted liposuction (UAL), power-assisted liposuction (PAL), radiofrequency-assisted liposuction (RFAL) and laser-assisted liposuction (LAL). These methods reduce operator fatigue and aid in the removal of particularly difficult or fibrous fat deposits, as in the cases of secondary liposuction. In addition, the LAL and RFAL literature claim fat destruction and skin tightening. All types of liposuction, with and without energy assistance, may be performed with a combination of tumescent anesthesia with or without general anesthesia or intravenous sedation. The demand for faster recovery, less downtime, and fear of traditional anesthesia has led to changes in patient perception and expectations where a gradual transition from hospital-based surgery under general anesthesia to office-based facilities utilizing minimally noninvasive techniques under local anesthesia have gained popularity. Liposuction, with or without energy assistance, under local anesthesia and oral medications alone has been proven to be a safe and effective alternative with a faster recuperation when compared with traditional methods of anesthesia and with a lower cost. For the body contouring aesthetic surgeon, the cornerstone of effective SAL under local anesthesia is the complete understanding of proper lidocaine dosing as well as its metabolism and risks of toxicity.

9.2 Preoperative Evaluation

The history and physical examination remains the same regardless of the method of anesthesia. A thorough review of systems with a focus on surgical history is conducted while also documenting any history of needle phobia and vaso-vagal episodes which would preclude the awake anesthesia option. In our experience, the actual number of true contraindications is very small once a thorough history is taken. Additionally, the patient tolerance to opioids and local anesthetics, chronic use of diuretics, or weight loss supplements will factor into the surgeon's decision to proceed under local anesthesia. All female patients of child-bearing age are checked for unexpected pregnancy. It is our practice to obtain basic screening laboratory values including a complete blood count (CBC), electrolyte panel, and coagulation studies. The physical examination focuses on the anatomic location and amount of adipose tissue to be resected and the assessment of the skin elasticity to determine the patient's candidacy for liposuction. It is notable that the anticipated volume of fat removal is no less when SAL is performed in the awake patient than in traditional anesthesia.

9.3 Preoperative Medications

Oral medications are given at least one half hour prior to the procedure and include an antibiotic (i.e., cephalexin 500 mg or ciprofloxacin 500 mg), diazepam 10–20 mg and a tablet of hydrocodone 5 mg with acetaminophen 300 mg. Intravenous access is not required and patients are instructed to eat a light meal prior to the procedure to prevent gastrointestinals upset from the oral medications. Patients are relaxed, able to follow commands and are fully conversant throughout the procedure.

9.4 Local Anesthesia Method

In order to maximize patient comfort, the methodology used in our practice differs from the traditional technique of tumescent infiltration in several key ways, most importantly in that the tumescent solution used has a higher concentration of lidocaine than typically found with tumescent solutions used with traditional methods of anesthesia. In the awake patient, it is critical that the experience is as painless as possible since the endpoint of tumescent infiltration is complete patient analgesia. Even with an excellent aesthetic outcome, if the patient only remembers a painful experience, the operation cannot be considered a success. The goal of the technique is complete analgesia.

9.4.1 Tumescent Solution

In the standard solution used most frequently in our practice, 1000 mg lidocaine, 12 mL sodium bicarbonate, and 1.5 mL of 1:1,000 epinephrine is added to one liter of Ringer's lactate. This results in a 0.1% concentration of lidocaine where 1 mL of solution contains 1 mg of lidocaine. We found that the small amount of sodium bicarbonate buffers the slight acidity of the solution to reduce tissue irritation and pain upon injection. The American Society of Plastic Surgeons recommends a maximum lidocaine load of 35 mg lidocaine per kg body weight. For a 70 kg patient, the recommended maximum lidocaine dose injected in the subcutaneous fat layer is 2,450 mg lidocaine (70 kg × 35 mg lidocaine/kg). With the 0.1% lidocaine solution we use, the calculation is straightforward: 2,450 mL of *solution* contains 2,450 mg of lidocaine. Therefore, the maximum *volume* of tumescent to be injected in a 70 kg patient is 2,450 mL.

Step One: Tumescent Infiltration

The access site is injected with 1% lidocaine with epinephrine and dilute sodium bicarbonate directly into the subcutaneous fat layer with a 30 gauge needle (▶Fig. 9.1). The needle is withdrawn slowly during injection so that the dermis is the last layer to be injected. Next, a 14 gauge hollow needle is used to create a circular access puncture point in the skin (▶Fig. 9.2). Stevens tenotomy scissors are used to carefully dilate the access to accommodate a 14 gauge Wells-Johnson blunt-tipped infiltration cannula (▶Fig. 9.3). We have found over time that these circular incisions tend to resist unintended widening of the incision and heal better aesthetically than linear incisions while still accommodating a variety of cannula sizes and diameters.

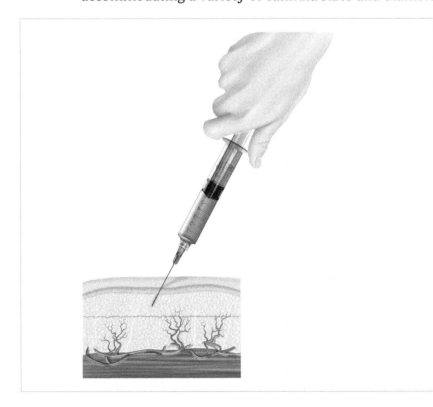

Fig. 9.1 Injection of the access point with 1% lidocaine with epinephrine.

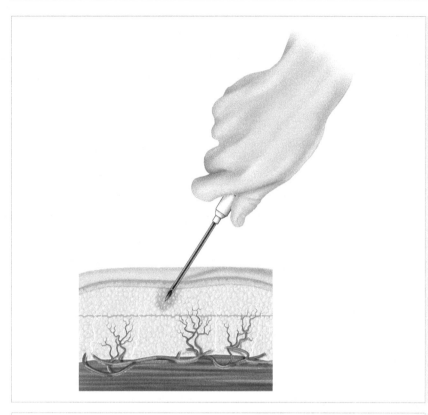

Fig. 9.2 A 14 gauge hollow needle used to create a circular access incision.

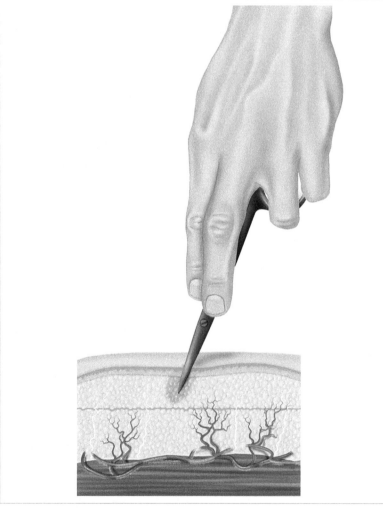

Fig. 9.3 A Stevens tenotomy scissors used to dilate the access incision to accommodate cannulas of varying diameters.

A 12–16 gauge blunt-tipped infiltration cannula (Wells-Johnson Corp., Tuscon, AZ), is introduced into the intermediate subcutaneous fat space and passed through the superficial fascial system (SFS) often with a palpable 'pop' until the tip lies just above the fascia of the muscle layer. This is done *without* injecting fluid. It has been our experience that the pain in this area is negligible most likely due to the paucity of nerve endings in this layer (▶ Fig. 9.4). Once the patient states that there is no pain at this point, infiltration of tumescent fluid begins at a slow rate of not more than 150–200 mL per minute (▶ Fig. 9.5). The cannula moves in small increments, allowing the hydrostatic pressure of the fluid to gradually fill the space until analgesia is achieved. Like a pebble dropped into calm waters, the ripples propagate in the same manner as the lidocaine diffuses throughout the treatment area.

Once the deepest layer is infiltrated, the cannula is withdrawn gradually while simultaneously injecting tumescent fluid into the more superficial layers (▶ Fig. 9.6). The last layer to be injected is the subdermal layer which has the greatest number of nerve endings and, hence, is the most sensitive layer. Care is taken to avoid peu d'orange as this is very painful and distorting of the anatomy without any benefit. This stage is complete once the patient confirms total analgesia.

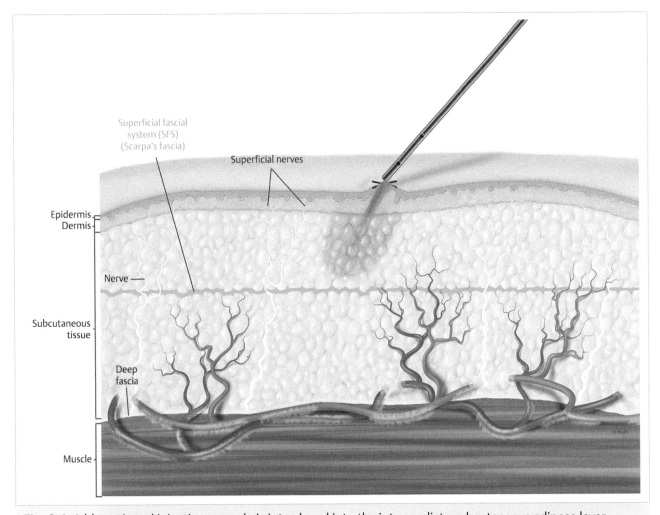

Fig. 9.4 A blunt-tipped injection cannula is introduced into the intermediate subcutaneous adipose layer.

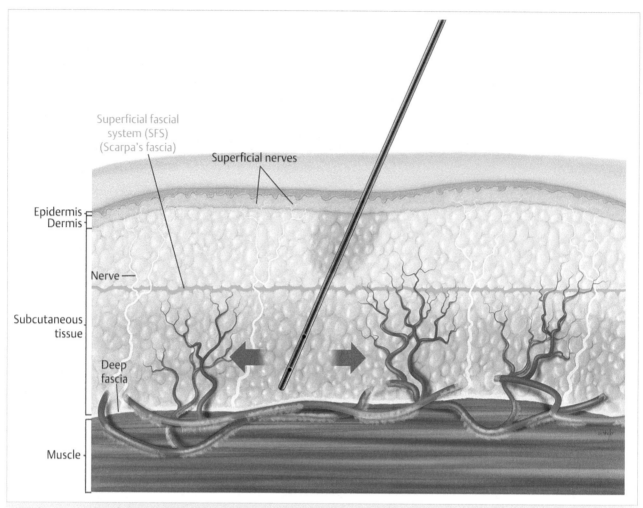

Fig. 9.5 The cannula is passed through the SFS with a palpable 'pop' before injecting tumescent fluid. Once above the fascia, the deep layer is injected with the fluid.

Step Two: Application of Laser Energy

In our practice, the SmartLipo™ Nd: Yag laser platform (Cynosure Corp., Westford, MA) was used to deliver 1440 nm wavelength laser energy into the subcutaneous fat through a 1000 micron diameter fiber-optic cable. Patient exclusion criteria include medical contraindications to liposuction and/or the medicines used, body mass index greater than 30, severe skin laxity, patient objection to an awake procedure, and unrealistic patient expectations. The same criteria used for traditional SAL are used to determine the adequacy of skin for LAL, which included the pinch test, presence or absence of dermal striae, and subjective determination of elasticity. The applied power setting is set maximally at 15.5 watts with a total energy application ranging from 2,000 to 24,000 joules per site. The fiberoptic cannula is placed in the deep and intermediate subcutaneous spaces while moving it at a rate of at least one cm/sec. The endpoint of laser energy deposition is when enough of the fat (a strong chromophore for the 1440 nm laser wavelength) becomes emulsified to cause a clinical easing of the passage of the instrument through the adipose tissue.

When a natural curvature in the anatomy, bony prominence, or other areas at risk of an "end hit" thermal injury is encountered, the laser would be intermittently switched off as needed to minimize the risk of a burn. For example, the neck in the hyperextended position warrants caution in the area of the

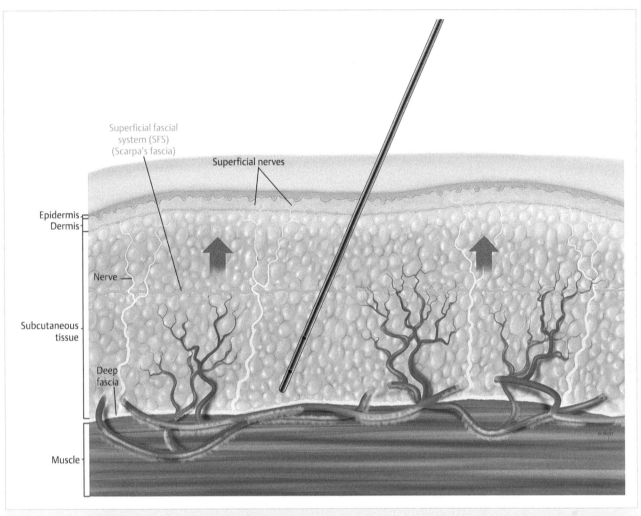

Fig. 9.6 The hydrostatic pressure of the infiltration allows gradual anesthetizing of the soft tissues toward the superficial fat layer and more nerve-rich subdermis.

midline. This area typically corresponds to the soft tissue just above the thyroid cartilage (▶ Fig. 9.7a, b). Suction assisted lipolysis is then performed using standard manual Mercedes-style tip liposuction cannulas and/or with 3.0 mm, 4.0 mm and 5.0 mm Mercedes-style tip PAL cannulas in the same subcutaneous planes. A closed suction drain is placed where a liter or more of total aspirate was removed to minimize the risk of seroma formation. All access incisions were closed with 5–0 nylon and the patients were placed in compression garments.

9.4.2 Intraoperative Considerations

Under local anesthesia, patients function as their own monitors regarding pain management and physiologic well-being. For example, if a patient exhibits an area of residual pain and sensitivity, it warrants injection of tumescent fluid to achieve total comfort. If the patient remains anxious during the case, additional oral medication can provide more comfort. It is critical to be in tune with every patient complaint or unexpected movement since it serves as an early warning system that the operating cannula might be in the wrong anatomic position. Only the dermal and subcutaneous fat planes have complete analgesia; mechanical violation of the fascia, muscular layers, and deeper

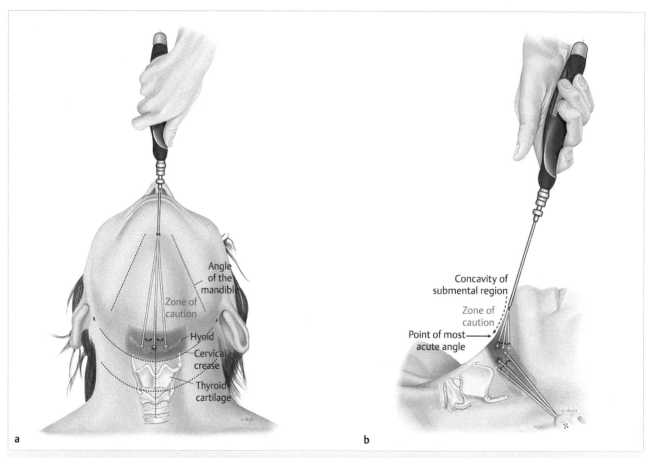

Fig. 9.7 (a, b) Taking into account areas of natural anatomic curves and overlapping of energy deposition is crucial to avoid 'end hits' of the laser energy and/or over-suctioning resulting in burns and contour deformities.

structures will elicit pain which the patient will immediately react to. This provides the operating surgeon excellent monitoring information lacking when general anesthesia is used where potentially catastrophic maneuvers can be avoided because of continuous patient feedback.

Another advantage of SAL in the awake patient is how easily and safely the patient is positioned. Aside from the fact that no additional personnel is required, it allows the patient to actively participate in his her care. Significantly, there is no need for an anesthesiologist and no airway maintenance concerns. Pressure points do not need to be specifically targeted with additional padding, and the overall time it takes to re-position the patient is measured in seconds, not minutes. The patient also benefits psychologically where the operation is perceived less threatening than surgery and more as a treatment. There is reduced operator fatigue as well.

From a thermoregulation standpoint, the awake patient maintains homeostasis with regard to body temperature and circulation. The room temperature is maintained according to patient preference. No anti-thrombotic protocols are necessary as there were no published reports of thrombo-embolic events in liposuction under local anesthesia known at the time of this publication. Muscle tone is normal and the patient can actively contract the underlying muscles if asked by the surgeon in order to outline the areas of fat removal in real-time as liposuction occurs that is impossible in the anesthetized patient.

From a fluid management perspective, the volume of tumescent fluid injected and hence the total volume of aspirate removed rarely exceeds

4 liters. The volume is limited by the lidocaine load which is carefully calculated according to patient body weight preoperatively as mentioned earlier. In our experience, no intravenous hydration was needed as the patients were typically fluid volume positive at the conclusion of the case from the tumescent injection and the overall volumes were modest. Patient demonstrated adequate oral hydration prior to discharge. If multiple areas were required for liposuction, the patient would be brought back in stages in order to maintain a safe range of lidocaine load as well as volume removal. Shorter recovery times have been seen with the local anesthesia option where return to daily activities typically occurred within 48 hours of the operation in the majority of patients.

Practice management advantages include reduced costs and staffing requirements with a single medical assistant. No anesthesiologist, nurse anesthetist, scrub nurse or recovery room nurse is required. Operating in an accredited, office-based surgical facility generally has lower fees when compared to hospitals and ambulatory surgical facilities. These factors increase patient acceptance and the local anesthesia technique may be extended into other body contouring procedures and presents a cost-effective management tool for small secondary procedures and/or staged procedures leading to better patient satisfaction.

9.5 Postoperative Considerations

Immediately following surgery, patients have complete analgesia for several hours due to the lidocaine effect. Patients are instructed to take one to two tablets of hydrocodone/acetaminophen prior to sleeping the first evening in anticipation of discomfort that occurs when the lidocaine is metabolized. All patients undergo early ambulation with few physical restrictions except avoidance of heavy exercise or running for at least 2 weeks postoperatively. Nylon sutures are removed at 10 days. Compression garments are worn for only 7–10 days. Patients then have the option to switch to commercially available compression workout gear afterwards for the next 2–3 weeks. Postoperative visits at 3, 6, and 12 months are routinely scheduled.

9.6 Complications

Unlike liposuction under general anesthesia, there were no published reports of pulmonary embolism or intra-abdominal organ perforation under local anesthesia. Minor complications are similar to traditional means of liposuction and include cellulitis, seromas, and hematomas. Regarding the energy-assisted liposuction modalities of laser, radiofrequency and ultrasound, minor burns and skin loss have been reported but were not correlated to the type of anesthesia used.

Specific to this technique, however, is the greater attention given to the possibility of lidocaine toxicity due to the higher relative amounts the awake patient requires. It has been reported by Samdal et al that larger doses of lidocaine and epinephrine in tumescent solution during SAL have earlier and higher concentration peaks in measured serum levels. Pitman et al reported doses as high as 63.8 mg/kg in his series of 142 patients with the highest recorded serum lidocaine level of 4.2 mcg/mL at 12 hours postoperatively. Although we report no adverse events in our series, further studies are warranted to assess absorption rates and peak serum levels at these higher lidocaine concentrations. Early signs and symptoms that the surgeon must be aware of include peri-oral numbness which may progress to nausea/vomiting, agitation, anxiety, etc. Early recognition is paramount.

Pearls

- Inject tumescent slowly and begin in the deep subcutaneous adipose layer in order to minimize pain on infiltration.
- The excellent safety profile and short recovery time are increasingly demanded by patients.
- No need for anesthesia services and multiple medical staff.
- Have the patient position him or herself with no need for DVT prophylaxis or heating blankets.
- Significant cost savings.

Pitfalls ✕

- Fewer total number of anatomic areas treatable in one session (lidocaine and volume limits).
- Learning curve to achieve reliable level of analgesia in the awake patient.
- Not all patients candidates (i.e., hyperanxiety).
- Slightly increased risk of lidocaine toxicity.

Suggested Readings

Apfelberg DB. Results of multicenter study of laser-assisted liposuction. Clin Plast Surg 1996; 23(4):713–719

Boeni R. Safety of tumescent liposuction under local anesthesia in a series of 4,380 patients. Dermatology 2011; 222(3):278–281

Chia CT, Theodorou SJ. 1,000 consecutive cases of laser-assisted liposuction and suction-assisted lipectomy managed with local anesthesia. Aesthetic Plast Surg 2012; 36(4):795–802

Katz BE, Bruck MC, Coleman WP, III. The benefits of powered liposuction versus traditional liposuction: a paired comparison analysis. Dermatol Surg 2001; 27(10):863–867

Klein JA. Tumescent technique for local anesthesia improves safety in large-volume liposuction. Plast Reconstr Surg 1993; 92(6):1085–1098, discussion 1099–1100

Scuderi N, Paolini G, Grippaudo FR, Tenna S. Comparative evaluation of traditional, ultrasonic, and pneumatic assisted lipoplasty: analysis of local and systemic effects, efficacy, and costs of these methods. Aesthetic Plast Surg 2000; 24(6):395–400

Teimourian B, Rogers WB, III. A national survey of complications associated with suction lipectomy: a comparative study. Plast Reconstr Surg 1989; 84(4):628–631

10 Radiofrequency-Assisted Liposuction for Body Contouring

Spero J. Theodorou, Christopher T. Chia, and Erez Dayan

Abstract

Body contouring has been addressed through liposuction alone or with skin excision procedures. Traditionally, only individuals with relatively mild skin excess could be managed with liposuction alone. There has long been a need for a technology that can safely and reproducibly tighten skin without lengthy incisions. Radiofrequency (RF) induced thermal contraction has been used in various medical and surgical specialties for many years but was only approved by the FDA in 2016 to assist in body contouring. The radiofrequency-assisted liposuction (RFAL) device Bodytite (Inmode, Ltd, Toronto, Canada) utilizes this effective technology to specifically heat the subcutaneous tissue and the skin in an effective, safe, and reproducible way. In this chapter, we offer an overview of the Bodytite device including the built-in safeguards, a guide to proper patient selection, and highlight the pearls and pitfalls of this exciting technology. RFAL is a powerful tool for thermal contraction of the soft tissues throughout the body in properly selected cases.

Keywords: Body contouring, liposuction, radiofrequency, radiofrequency-assisted liposuction, RFAL

10.1 Radiofrequency Technology

Liposuction has increasingly become the most sought after body contouring procedure internationally. However, the goal of achieving concomitant skin tightening in liposuction has been elusive at best. The need for a device that can accomplish tissue heating in a safe and reproducible way leading to skin contraction without lengthy incisions can have immeasurable benefits to patients. The use of RF was initially reported in the literature as a noninvasive device. It has led to the use of RF as an energy-based platform for body contouring with FDA approval in 2016.

The elusive goal of achieving skin tightening in liposuction has been attempted with laser assisted liposuction (LAL).[1] Paul et al introduced RFAL technology in 2009 and showed linear contraction at 12 months of up to 47%.[2,3] Unlike laser liposuction the focus of the energy is not directed at the dermis per say but at a deeper level. The ability to heat and treat large volumes of tissue, due to RF's ability to be utilized in the subcutaneous and deep adipose tissue without compromising skin safety, has been the mainstay of RFAL technology. This process of thermal enhanced remodeling of the soft tissue leading to skin tightening has led to the use of RFAL in patients who would otherwise be marginal or poor candidates for traditional liposuction techniques.

10.2 RFAL: Mechanism of Action

RF thermal-induced contraction has been described in medicine in various applications such as vein ablation, orthopedics, and ophthalmology.

Contraction of the collagen fibers occurs at different temperatures depending on the type of collagen. The optimal temperature for collagen contracture has been reported to be 60–80°C.[4] This contraction does not necessarily cause connective tissue damage but instead induces a restructuring effect of the collagen fiber framework. Once the tissue reaches the threshold temperature it immediately undergoes contraction in a dramatic fashion. This effect has been described in studies of the cornea, cartilage, and vascular tissue in the past. RF energy is applied internally directly to the deep adipose and subcutaneous tissue with lower heat levels applied to the dermis. This results in tissue contraction that occurs mainly due to the contribution of deeper adipo-fascial layers. Specifically, heating of the Fibro-Septal Network (FSN) leads to dermal contraction (▶Fig. 10.1).

The target temperature at which soft tissue matrix contracture optimally occurs is 38–42°C.[5] The internal measured temperature can range from 55–70°C however this is only relevant as it relates to the external temperature reading. In other words, the endpoint of 38–42°C measured externally should be reached in order to achieve the desired result of dermal tightening.

10.3 RF Device

The RFAL device Bodytite (Inmode, Ltd, Toronto, Canada) consists of a handpiece with two electrodes attached to an RF power source (▶Fig. 10.2). The internal electrode is coated with a Teflon tip in order to avoid end hit injuries. It has a conductive tip that emits RF energy that flows between the internal electrode and the external electrode which in turn overlies the surface of the skin. An energy field is thus created between the two electrodes that

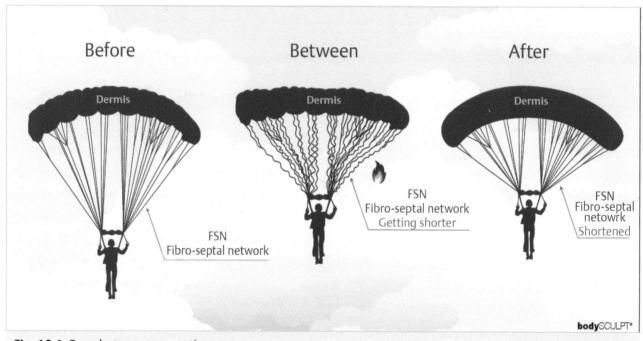

Fig. 10.1 Parachute + cross-section.

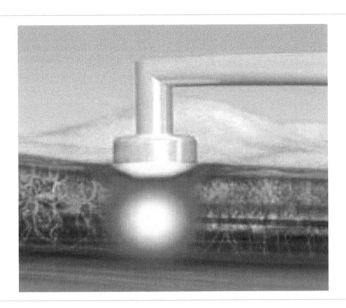

Fig. 10.2 RFAL device, Bodytite.

translates into a thermal effect on the interposed tissues. Once the area to be treated is tumesced the internal probe is inserted and is passed back and forth in smooth liposuction-like strokes. At the same time the external probe glides in tandem along the surface of the skin. The skin has been prepped with sterile ultrasound gel in order to minimize interference and facilitate movement of the external electrode.

The subcutaneous tissue between the two probes is heated accordingly. The treated tissue tends to be hotter at the tip of the probe and recedes in temperature as it approaches the handle.

The depth of the internal probe is controlled by a wheel on the device that increases or decreases the distance between the two electrodes giving it a caliper-like appearance. The larger the distance between the two electrodes the larger amount of tissue is "sandwiched" between them resulting in a larger area heated.

The process of heating the tissues begins deep just like in liposuction. The difference being though, that instead of "debulking" the operator is heating. The movement of the probe is identical to the stroke of a liposuction cannula. In other words, deliberate and methodical with care not to spend too much time in one area. As heating progresses and the operator begins to treat the more superficial tissue he or she will be adjusting the wheel to close the distance between the two probes. As the surgeon approaches the dermis the distance between the electrodes is shortened even more in order to address the more superficial layers of the treated area. At no point does the internal probe come into contact with the under surface of the dermis or the subdermal plexus of nerves and vessels.

In conclusion the RF handpiece coagulates the adipose and connective tissue as well as the deep vasculature via the internal probe. The heating of the dermis occurs internally just below the external probe. The heating of the treated tissue block is homogenous and uniform (▶Fig. 10.3). Once the target temperature of 38–42°C is achieved the operator maintains the heat in that area for 1–3 min for optimal results.

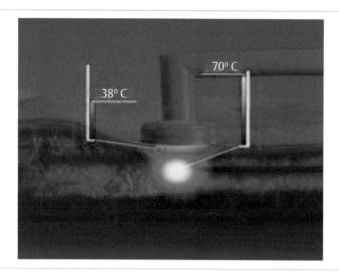

Fig. 10.3 The RFAL device Bodytite with two electrodes showing differential heating of the internal and external probe. The internal probe targets adipose, connective tissue, and the deep vasculature. The external probe heats the dermis.

The operator can then switch to a standard suction-assisted lipectomy (SAL) or power-assisted liposuction device (MicroAire, Charlottesville, VA, USA) to address the contouring aspect of the operation and bring the case to conclusion.

10.4 Safety Parameters

- The bodytite device has an audible bell that serves the purpose of warning the operator of the impending target goal temperature. As the target temperature of 38–42°C is reached, the bell sound intervals become shorter in duration warning the operator of the impending endpoint. This has the advantage of allowing the surgeon to focus on the operating field without needing to look at the LED screen for target temperature verification.
- The bodytite handpiece's internal probe has an infra-red thermistor which shuts down the energy output if the temperature exceeds predetermined parameters set before the onset of the case. For example the internal probe temperature can be set between 50–70°C and the external at 40°C depending on what the operator seeks to achieve.
- The teflon coated tip of the internal probe helps avoid end hit damage that can occur with any energy generating device in liposuction. However, the operator should be cognizant of this and avoid contact with the dermis by knowing where the tip is at all times (▶ Fig. 10.4).
- Any device that uses energy has the potential to cause peri-portal burns to the skin. Liberal application of petroleum-based ointment by the operator to the portal site in addition to constant movement of the bodytite handpiece can prevent this sort of injury from occurring. In addition the teflon coating of the internal probe protects the surrounding access point on the skin.
- Do not spend more time than 1–3 minutes in a given area once target temperature is achieved. Slow and continuous application of heat results in even heating of tissues resulting in a uniform result. Tissue response and patient tolerance are thus achieved[6] (▶ Fig. 10.5).

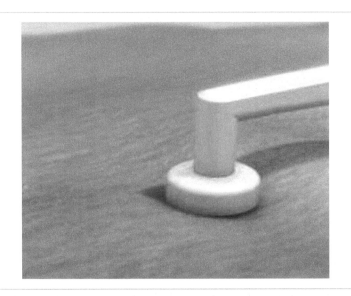

Fig. 10.4 The Bodytite external probe (shown), should remain in contact with the skin so that the internal probe (below the skin) remains deep enough to avoid burns to the skin. This device has other built in safeguards including a teflon coated tip to avoid end hit damage and potential burns to the skin.

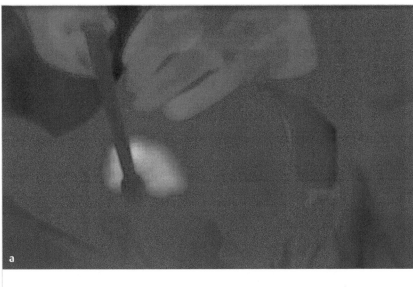

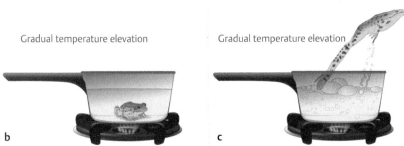

Gradual temperature elevation   Gradual temperature elevation

Fig. 10.5 These diagrams are an analogy for tissue response to higher energy settings (70 W and 38–42°C) used in previous studies with the radio frequency-assisted liposuction (RFAL) device and to the lower energy settings (35–40 W and 38–42°C) **(a)**. In our experience, both patient tolerance and tissue response to the energy delivered by the RFAL device are better at the lower energy settings as long as the same target temperature of 38–42°C is achieved. For tissue response to energy settings we use the analogy of a frog gradually being heated in a pot of water to a target temperature of 100°C **(b)** as opposed to the frog being placed in a pot of boiling water **(c)**. In the first instance, the frog (tissue response) tolerates the gradual increase in temperature and remains in the pot. In the second instance, the frog (tissue response) jumps out.

10.5 RFAL: Patient Selection

RFAL liposuction is ideal for a number of different scenarios. It should not be viewed as a substitute for traditional liposuction. Instead it fills a treatment efficacy gap where current technologies and methodology are lacking in their ability to contract skin. Refer to sections 10.5.1 and 10.5.2 for such examples.

10.5.1 RFAL Candidates

- Patients that are poor candidates for liposuction and not bad enough for an excisional procedure. This is a very large sub category of patients that have been turned down in the past for lack of effective treatment solutions (▶ Fig. 10.6a–h).

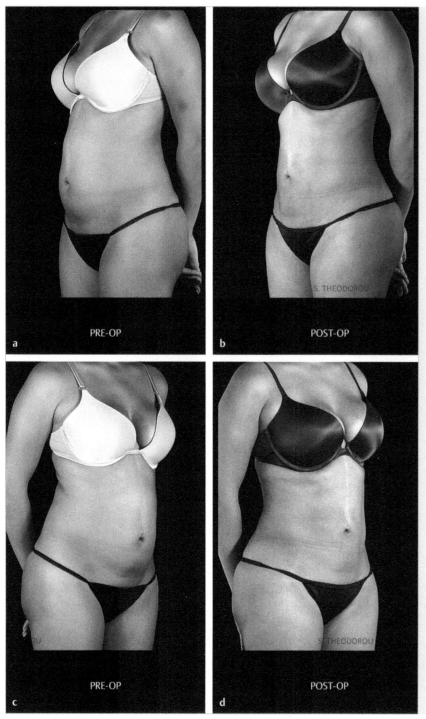

PRE-OP

POST-OP

PRE-OP

POST-OP

Fig. 10.6 A 30-year-old female. 35 watts 38°T. 2.7 LT. 48.8 KJ. 1 year. **(a, c, e, g)** Preoperative. **(b, d, f, h)** Postoperative.

(Continued)

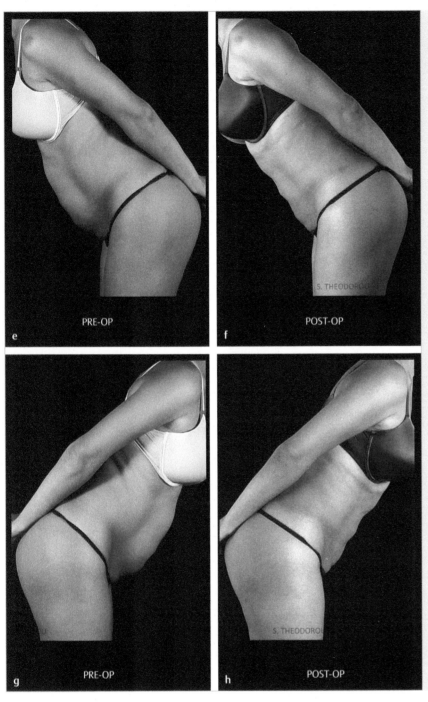

Fig. 10.6 (*Continued*) A 30-year-old female. 35 watts 38°T. 2.7 LT. 48.8 KJ. 1 year. (**a, c, e, g**) Preoperative. (**b, d, f, h**) Postoperative.

- Areas of non-adherence such as the arms. There is a very large number of patients with complaints of arm lipodystrophy and laxity that do not proceed with a brachioplasty operation due to the nature and the length of the scar.
- Medial thighs are good candidates for RFAL. This area is notorious for a high number of post-liposuction iatrogenic deformities. This occurs most commonly due to contour deformities related to laxity in this area.

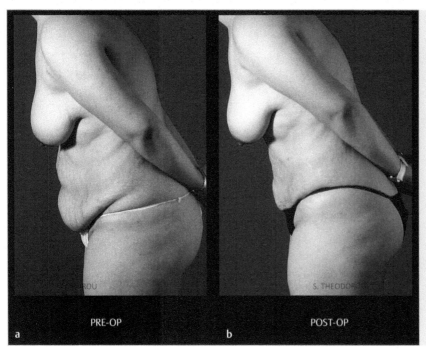

PRE-OP

a

POST-OP

b

Fig. 10.7 A 32-year-old female. 40 watts 40°T. 1.15LT. 53.1 KJ. 18 months. (a) Preoperative. (b) Postoperative.

- Female patients that have had children but are not candidates for an abdominoplasty due to minimal or moderate laxity of the skin and lack of a significant rectus diastasis. The laxity tends to occur mostly in the infa-umbilical area where the majority of the growth of the uterus occurs during pregnancy (►Fig. 10.7).
- Neck Laxity: Example such as middle age males not bad enough for a neck lift and not good candidates for liposuction (►Fig. 10.8a–h).

10.5.2 Poor RFAL Candidates

- Patients that are candidates for excisional procedures.
- Massive weight loss patients. The dermis is typically irreversibly damaged in these patients and as a result does not contract well or evenly.
- Patients with no adiposity. RFAL requires an intact fibro septal network (FSN) with fat to work best. As an example massive weight loss patients with a 'deflated' appearance and thin adipose tissue respond poorly to RFAL.
- Supra-umbilical skin overhang with no adiposity with or without striae.
- Patients with Fitzpatrick I–II over 50 years of age tend to have a mediocre to poor response when performing RFAL on the body. Same age patients that are Fitzpatrick III–IV respond much better to RF energy as a result of a thicker and more contractile dermis.

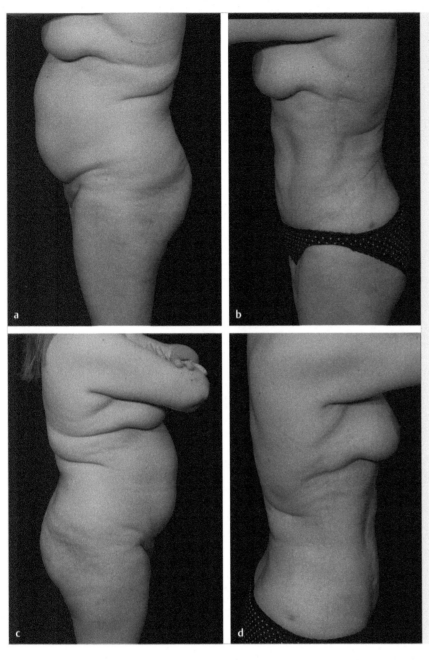

Fig. 10.8 (**a–d**) A 56-year-old female with Bodytite of the abdomen and flanks. 40 watts. Temperature 40.0°C and 70.0°C . 2019.

10.6 Pearls and Pitfalls

Pearls **M!**

- New treatment option that previously was not available to patients that are otherwise not candidates for liposuction due to skin laxity.
- RF technology is a great alternative to brachioplasty in many cases.
- RF allows surgeons to address laxity in the medial thighs more aggressively than previously possible since the RF energy will assist in the tightening (►Fig. 10.9).
- RF treats patient with neck laxity who are not candidates for neck or face lift.
- Abdominal laxity not bad enough for an abdominoplasty and ideal for liposuction (►Fig. 10.10).

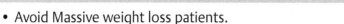

Pitfalls ✕

- Avoid Massive weight loss patients.
- Fitzpatrick I–II over 50 years of age.
- Avoid patients with striae.
- Thermal injury due to end hits and portal burns.
- Avoid patients that are candidates for excisional surgery.

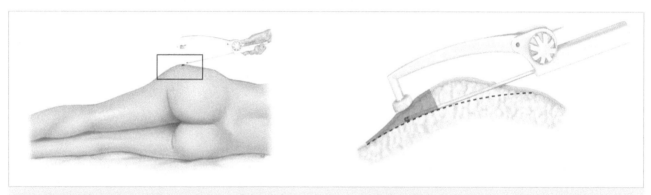

Fig. 10.9 A depiction of the convexity of the lateral thigh treatment zone in relationship to the straight BodyTite handpiece. Caution needs to be exercised in the type of convex treatment area in order to avoid end hits (direct injury) and a rapid increase in temperature that can lead to possible full thickness injury of the dermis (indirect injury). The top picture points out the area of treatment and the lower depicts the magnified area of interest. The area in red is the zone of caution.

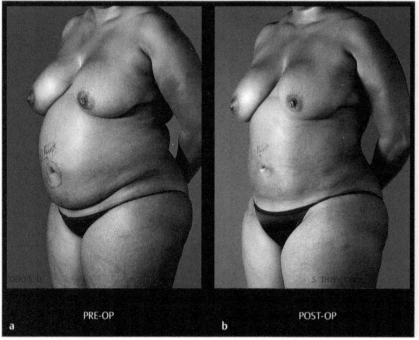

PRE-OP   POST-OP

a   b

Fig. 10.10 A 41-year-old female. 70 watts 40°T. 3.5LT. 103.8 KJ. WL30 13 months. **(a)** Preoperative. **(b)** Postoperative.

References

[1] Sasaki GH, Tevez A. Laser-assisted liposuction for facial and body contouring and tissue tightening: a 2-year experience with 75 consecutive patients. Semin Cutan Med Surg 2009;28(4):226–235

[2] Paul M, Mulholland RS. A new approach for adipose tissue treatment and body contouring using radiofrequency-assisted liposuction. Aesthetic Plast Surg 2009;33(5):687–694

[3] Chia CT, Neinstein RM, Theodorou SJ. Evidence-Based Medicine: Liposuction. Plast Reconstr Surg 2017;139(1):267e–274e

[4] Teruya TH, Ballard JL. New approaches for the treatment of varicose veins. Surg Clin North Am 2004;84(5):1397–1417, viii–ix

[5] Paul M, Blugerman G, Kreindel M, Mulholland RS. Three-dimensional radiofrequency tissue tightening: a proposed mechanism and applications for body contouring. Aesthetic Plast Surg 2011;35(1):87–95

[6] Theodorou SJ, Paresi RJ, Chia CT. Radiofrequency-assisted liposuction device for body contouring: 97 patients under local anesthesia. Aesthetic Plast Surg 2012;36(4):767–779

11 VASER Technology for Body Contouring

Alfredo Hoyos and Mauricio Perez

Abstract

Ultrasound technologies were introduced to liposuction in the late 80s to selectively emulsificate the adipose tissue and facilitate the fat extraction. Three generations of devices has been developed reducing the amount of required energy while maintaining the emulsification efficacy. It works by creating a vibration frequency close to the fat specific resonance which disrupts the fat cells while safely avoid the surrounding tissues. The use of different type of probes and energy intensity allows to treat different conditions and types of patients. The ultrasound also effects on the dermis by inducing retraction and reducing the amount of blood loss. The harvested fat has been successfully used for grafting due to the adequate viability.

The use of this technology requires an adequate training and safety protocol to achieve the desired results and avoid complications.

Keywords: Ultrasound, VASER, emulsification, resonance, high definition

Key Points

- Surgical specialties have always been susceptible of multiple technological innovations, since improvements in techniques and results are almost always associated with new devices or gadgets. Body contour surgery is one of a kind in this matter, as many devices do exist as techniques for liposuction. One of the best devices for this purpose is vibration amplification of sound energy at resonance(VASER), which is crucial to perform high definition lipoplasty.
- VASER uses ultrasound energy to emulsify adipose tissue and improves fat removal without vascular or cell injury.
- Two different modes (continuous and pulsed) are employed depending on the zone to treat and the type of procedure you would like to perform.
- Ancillary procedures can be used in addition to VASER-assisted lipoplasty depending on the surgeon's preferences and type of surgery.
- Different probes and cannulas have been designed to help the surgeon perform a safer procedure with less morbidity and better results.
- VASER-assisted body contour surgery has been widely performed with low morbidity and low rate of complications.

11.1 Introduction

11.1.1 Ultrasonic Technology in Medicine, History, Uses, and Refinements

New technologies and devices have positively impacted the outcomes and the way liposuction is performed. Ultrasound is a powerful tool both for diagnosis and treatment in many medical conditions. Studied since 1930s for therapeutic and diagnostic usage, the first applications were applied for the heating capacity to produce a biological effect. The devices rapidly improve in such a way that it was even able to be successfully used for vestibular nerve destruction in Meniere's disease and even brain tissue ablation in Parkinson's disease.

Kelman introduced phaco emulsification for cataracts in 1967 after being inspired by his dentist's ultrasound device for descaling. Also, neurosurgeons started using it for selective destruction of tumors, and general surgeons for cutting and coagulating tissues during laparoscopic surgery. In the late 1980s and early 1990s, Scuderi and Zocchi pioneered the application of ultrasound for selective emulsification and removal of fat for body contouring. Ultrasound devices have been upgraded by 3 generations and nowadays we regard the latest technology with specific targeted tissues depending on the device physics and specifications. In 2001, Sound Surgical Technologies introduced a third-generation device, designed to improve safety by reducing the power delivered to the tissues whilst maintaining efficacy. This new technology was patented by the name VASER that became swiftly the gold standard for high-definition body sculpting surgery.

By including VASER to body contour liposculpture, tissues were highly protected from burns, intraoperative and postoperative bleeding decreased, and stem-cell harvesting was possible from the extracted adipose tissue, with the aim to be grafted later in surgery in some areas with lack of volume or projection. Different studies have been published supporting the use of ultrasound in cosmetic surgery and VASER is not the exception. However, it has been proposed for many other uses including dental cleansing, physiotherapy and so forth. Currently, the FDA has approved ultrasound therapy for cancer, gynecologic ablations, glaucoma, laparoscopic surgery, kidney stone comminution, plantar fasciitis, phaco-emulsification, thrombus dissolution, transdermal drug delivery, bone fracture healing, and lately for skin tightening and adipose tissue removal. All these indications has some evidence to consider them useful and safe for human use (▶ Fig. 11.1).

Although, VASER-assisted lipoplasty typically takes longer than standard suction-assisted lipoplasty due to the extra step required for emulsification of adipose tissue before aspiration, the technology has several advantages. Fine

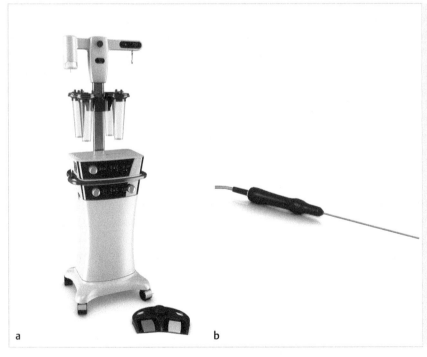

a   b

Fig. 11.1 VASER system: ultrasonic electric generator **(a)** and handpiece **(b)**.

probes and tunable power allow delicate and superficial tissues to be treated without causing unwanted irregularities. The unique pulsed (VASER) mode also halves the energy delivered to the tissues and represents an important feature for subdermal clearance of fat without causing complications. In order to treat fibrous tissue such as the back or male breasts, the power output is increased, continuous ultrasound is selected, and a more aggressive probe is selected. The cavitation and mechanical forces that are produced with the VASER probes vibrating at ultrasonic frequencies disrupt relatively weak adipose tissue much more readily than more dense tissue such as vessels, nerves, and fibrous septae. As a result, there is a selective emulsification of fat with sparing of surrounding tissues. This translates to less bleeding, less bruising, and an easier and more rapid recovery for the patient than suction-assisted lipoplasty. The majority of fat aspirated following treatment with VASER is viable. This is particularly important for high-definition body sculpting where large volumes of fat grafts may be used to contour the buttocks, hips, or breasts.

Consequently, this technology allowed the surgeon to perform better procedures, with less complications and for sure, a new era of body sculpting was ahead. In the next paragraphs we will explain deeply about VASER and its benefits, but focusing on its use in high definition body sculpting.

11.1.2 VASER Physics: How it Works?

VASER technology is somehow different from previous generations of ultrasound as we discussed above. The main difference compared to other devices is the way the energy is delivered to the tissues: not just ultrasound but **resonance**. This is a physical effect seen in nature and many other disciplines rather than electronics. This concept is based in two notions: one is that the frequency of the device (36 mHz) is closest to the resonance of fat. While fat vibrates, it gets emulsified with less power delivered. The second notion is the cell size: comparatively, fat cells are 10 times bigger than other cells around (blood vessels, nerves, connective tissue), making fat more sensitive to the ultrasonic energy than the other tissues.

Most ultrasound surgical instruments oscillate or vibrate between 20 kHz and 60 kHz. VASER employs probes that oscillate 36,000 times per second as we mentioned before, so its technology allows safe and efficient emulsification of fat in all subcutaneous layers, including the superficial subdermal layer, preserving as much of the tissue matrix as possible, yet still remove the desired amount of fatty tissue. They designed smaller diameter solid probes (2.2–4.5 mm) and a unique grooved tip design to emulsify fat efficiently at 36 kHz, but also preserving surrounding tissues and structures. The correct application and treatment with VASER enables smooth, even results and optimizes postoperative skin retraction. This device is also an excellent tool to facilitate fat harvesting, stem cell decantation and then grafting during the body contouring procedure.

Consequently, the therapeutic effect has a thermal and a non thermal mechanism depending on the interaction of the wave with the tissue. Cavitation occurs when there is enough air in the tissue where bubbles are created, vibrate and oscillate around an equilibrium ratio which produces high pressures and high temperature. The acoustic radiation happens when the momentum is transferred from the sound field to the object (▶ Fig. 11.2).

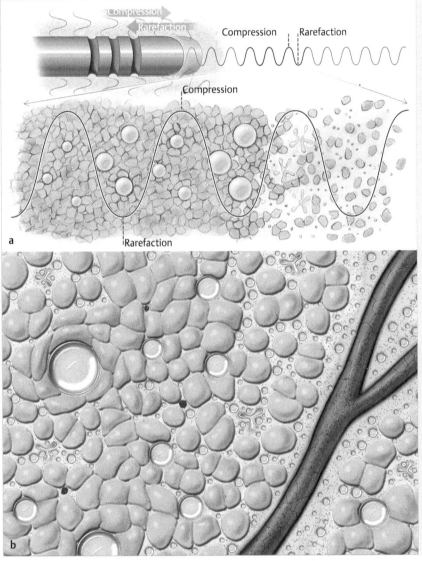

Fig. 11.2 Fat emulsification: VASER system gets advantage of ultrasound energy and vibration to disrupt the adipose supporting tissue **(a)**. Compression over the fatty tissue through vibrating ultrasound energy and the rarefaction that is pulled back allows the adipose cell liberation from the connective tissue. This will allow easier and safer fat extraction without injuring noble structures **(b)**.

11.1.3 Indications for VASER

The third-generation ultrasound console consists of an integrated system including all the elements required for flow rate-controlled tumescent infiltration, tissue-selective destruction of fat, negative pressure aspiration, and collection of emulsified fat in disposable canisters. Foot pedals control infiltration and ultrasound delivery, and dials on the digital display component adjust flow rate and ultrasound power output. The amplitude of energy can be adjusted at the console, by 10% increments, from 0 to 100%. The VASER system comprises an electronic generator and an ultrasonic handpiece. Within it, the electric energy is converted to mechanical energy in the form of vibration through a piezoelectric transducer. This vibratory motion is channeled through the handler to the attached titanium probe. As such, the metal probe is made to vibrate at 36 kHz (ultrasonic frequency), at which probes of certain lengths vibrate longitudinally with the handpiece. The forward and back movement of the probe is maximal at the tip where energy is focused. Although the displacement of the tip of the probe is only in the order of microns, it is sufficiently powerful to exhibit its effects on the surrounding tissues. The solid titanium probes are attached to the ultrasonic handpiece using an attachable wrench to ensure a snug fit. The probes are used to emulsify fat in an extra step before aspiration, thus preserving the fluid medium required to protect tissues from excessive ultrasound energy.

Subsequently, by increasing the amplitude on the generator (10–100%), the displacement becomes greater and the power increases. Tissue interaction between titanium ultrasonic probes and wet adipose tissue that leads to disruption and emulsification can be broadly divided into three mechanisms: cavitation, mechanical, and thermal. Mechanical disruption of fat occurs at the tip of the probe, where the vibrating metal surface comes in contact with the adipocytes. As we know, vibrating and moving energy is lost by heat at the tip of the probe, so it must be constantly moving within the tissues in order to avoid the incidence of burns and seroma. Cavitation and mechanical disruption of adipose tissue occurs due to the relative fragility of this tissue compared to other tissues such as vessels, muscle, and nerves.

11.1.4 Continuous versus Pulsed Mode: Energy Release and Heat Conversion

The ultrasonic devices were initially designed to continuously deliver the energy to the tissue as the standard mechanism to achieve a biological effect. By this means the total amount of energy and the heat produced is also higher like the side effects. Previous ultrasound systems delivered energy to the tissues continuously once activated. With new devices, the option to deliver energy continuously or in a pulsed mode (VASER) is available.

Pulsed mode delivers 10 bursts of energy per second, roughly halving the total energy delivered to the tissues while maintaining efficiency. This mode is utilized in delicate areas or during high definition work very close to the dermis. In a similar fashion, specific cannulas were designed to use with VASER and have smaller portholes than standard liposuction ones of the same diameters. This feature reduces avulsion and trauma to tissues during the aspiration of emulsified fat. A small hole in the handpiece of the aspiration cannula ensures that there is constant flow of aspirate through the tubing, even when the cannula is in the patient. The venting through the cannula reduces the vacuum and reduces trauma to the tissues.

11.1.5 Probe Design and Use

One of the main advantages of the VASER system relates to its safety, smoothness, and ability to treat the superficial tissues. First of all, solid probes are used so the protective tumescent fluid is not withdrawn during ultrasound delivery to the tissues. Ultrasound energy should never be delivered to dry tissues. In the same way, the probes are smaller in diameter compared to their predecessors. Since the amount of energy delivered to tissues is approximately proportional to the square of the diameter of the probe, narrower probes deliver much less energy and are safer. The efficiency of the narrower VASER probes are not just preserved but increased due to the grooves at the tip of the probes. The grooves increase surface area and increase coupling with the surrounding tissues. Cavitation occurs in front of as well as to the sides of the grooved tip, increasing efficiency and reducing the amount of total energy required to disrupt a given volume of adipose tissue.

The probes play an important role in the way the energy is efficiently administered to the tissues. They are 2.2, 2.9, 3.7, and 4.5 mm in diameter.

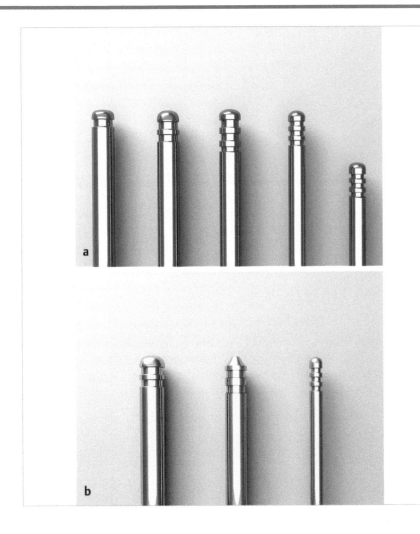

Fig. 11.3 Probes and tips: Round tips are preferred for first-time procedures, grooves determine the radial energy reach **(a)**. Special tips are preferred for secondary procedures or excess fibrotic vs fat tissue **(b)**.

The tip has a variable configuration of grooves in such an arrangement, that ultrasound energy is delivered both from the tip and from the sides of the probe in varying ratios depending on whether a one, two, or three-grooved probe is used. The 2.2 mm probe is used for facial applications and the others for body applications depending on volume of tissue treated.

The appropriate probe size is selected proportional to the volume of tissue. The grooved-probe design improves efficiency of emulsification of fatty tissues using less energy than would be required with previous instruments. Fewer tip grooves are used for disrupting fat immersed in fibrous areas. Probes with more grooves are helpful for debulking softer fat. There are some specialized probes for particular tasks like cellulite and gynecomastia management (▶Fig. 11.3).

11.1.6 VASER–Assisted Lipoplasty (VAL)

Indications and advantages (secondary liposuction, fibrosis, obese patients).

Wide research attempts looking for evidence about the advantages and disadvantages in the clinical setting has let aside the mere speculation to a clear scientific statement. The current literature supports ultrasound in cosmetic surgery in many fields. The VASER technology has supporting high quality evidence demonstrating its safety profile, the fat removal effectiveness, and the harvested fat viability among others.

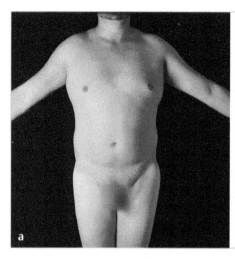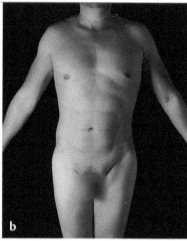

Fig. 11.4 VASER high definition lipoplasty, performed in a 38-year-old man. Note the difference in the abundant fat pad in the preoperative **(a)** picture and the new muscular body contour in the 6-month postoperative **(b)** picture.

Compared to the traditional suction-assisted lipoplasty, when using ultrasound emulsification the skin retraction is improved, the blood loss is significantly reduced as well as the physical effort needed for the extraction. This is especially true when highly fibrotic tissue is approached like in secondary procedures where the expected healing mechanisms create large fibrous septae. In those cases, the surgeon's physical effort and the blood loss is significantly increased, as well as the rate of fat extraction is reduced. This scenario makes ultrasound devices an essential tool to reduce bleeding rates, improve outcomes and of course let the surgeon perform a more comfortable procedure. In order to treat fibrous tissue, like the posterior torso or the male breasts, the power output needs to be increased in continuous mode and a more aggressive probe, like the one-grooved or arrow probe, is selected (▶Fig. 11.4).

11.1.7 VASER Skin Retraction

VAL is performed as a 3-step procedure: Infiltration, Emulsification and Aspiration. The traditional tumescent technique is used for infiltration, soon after that emulsification takes place. Ultrasound energy delivered to the tissues is selective for lobules of fat bathed in tumescent solution, such that collateral damage to the tissue matrix, lymphatics, nerves, and vessels is minimized. The ability to halve energy delivered to the tissues using the pulsed mode is important during the very superficial work required for high definition lipoplasty, a procedure mastered by the authors where specific definition of the natural underlying anatomy is made through the entire body to get natural and athletic results in lipoplasty. Furthermore, the unique vented cannulas and small port holes facilitate refined contouring in delicate and superficial tissues and reduce avulsion and trauma to tissues. Therefore, ultrasound-assisted liposculpture has shown to reduce blood loss and improve skin retraction compared to suction-assisted lipoplasty. This premise is the basis of high-definition body contour surgery, as large surface areas are often treated in a single procedure and also controlled skin retraction is essential in order to reveal underlying muscular anatomy (▶Fig. 11.5).

Nagy and Vanek did a contralateral study in patients undergoing lipoplasty over the abdominal area. On one side traditional liposuction and on the other side VASER liposuction were performed. The degree of skin retraction was

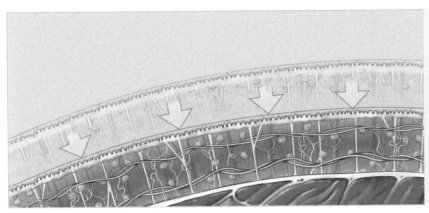

Fig. 11.5 Skin retraction. By removing fat in the superficial and deep layers, elastic properties of the skin and the compression over the underlying structures will end up in a new body contour.

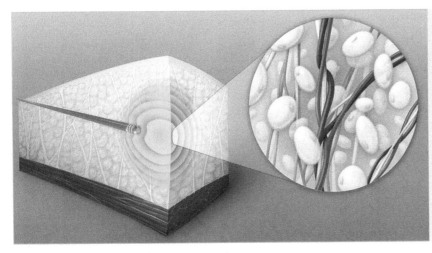

Fig. 11.6 VASER ultrasound energy used to cleave the fat connective tissue vibrates at a specific resonance in order to avoid noble structure lesions.

measured by UV ink: An statistically significant difference on the skin retraction was better achieved by VASER rather than traditional lipoplasty.

11.1.8 Blood Loss and VASER

A safe amount of fat removal is closely related to the admissible blood loss, the volume of infiltrated fluids and the surgical time. Cavitation produced with VASER probes disrupts the relatively weak adipose tissue more directly than a dense tissue like vessels, nerves, and fibrous septae. It creates a selective emulsification of fat sparing the surrounding tissues. By reducing the blood loss and facilitating the surgeon's work, a larger amount of fat can be safely removed, then allowing this technique to be used in overweight and obese patients. Some publications support that bleeding might be reduced 4 to 5 times using VASER devices compared to traditional liposuction. Moreover, some studies performed in lipectomy flaps comparing VASER versus non-VASER liposuction have shown that VASER proved to be a better determinant for flap viability due to the subdermal vascular plexus preservation. These factors allow us to perform wider liposuction over lipectomy flaps and also achieve high definition lipoplasty over the flap (▶ Fig. 11.6).

11.1.9 Cell Viability After Use of VASER Liposuction

First-generation ultrasound devices used a high amount of energy that violently disrupt most of the adipose cell membranes and the stroma, resulting in poor fat viability and so an inadequate source of fat for grafting. The new development of a precise instrument that delivers the righteous amount of energy to emulsify but also to allow the cell survival was the key of the VASER system. Shaffer et al. demonstrated the metabolic activity of the adipocytes after the harvesting using a third-generation ultrasound and its suitability for grafting in an *in vitro* work. In our experience, fat harvesting by VASER and large-volume fat grafting have shown adequate integration and survival rates, however medical literature is still controversial in how the best harvesting method and fat graft preparation should be regarding liposuction. Some authors prefer decantation systems while immune tests and/or centrifugation remain the best choice for others.

11.1.10 Probes and Setting According to Each Patient

The delicate differences of the fat structure arrangement in the different anatomical areas and the desirable fat disposition according to gender and the cultural ideals is the basic knowledge required to choose the required energy and the type of probe tip. Great-diameter probes are preferred for deep and abundant debulking, while thinner ones are ideal for superficial framing and smooth definition. Curved cannulas are also designed to reach some anatomic zones to avoid additional incisions and perform a safer procedure. For patients with previous contour surgery smaller probes and pointed ones are desirable to liberate and disrupt fibrosis.

11.2 Complications

11.2.1 Prevention and Treatment

VASER proper use relies on several factors, so we must take advice of the unique properties of the system in order to avoid complications. The first one is the proper and sufficient infiltration of the tissue to be treated. Superficial and deep layers must be infiltrated separately, starting from the bottom towards the surface, in order to prevent burns due to the lack of fluid. A second factor should be the timing to use the ultrasonic power: VASER emulsification must be conducted for 1 or 2 minutes per each 100 mL of infiltration. The third factor is the VASER mode and power according to the layer: **pulsed** mode should be used in the superficial layer while **continuous** mode is reserved for the deep layers (avoid its use in the superficial). Different anatomical areas also require a different time, power, and even a different tool or probe. The energy required for the fat emulsification and the suction technique generates enough heat to produce burns which accounts for most complications associated with the ultrasound-assisted lipoplasty. Effort must be directed to strategies and techniques to avoid or reduce the risk of burning (▶Fig. 11.7).

Burns can be divided according to the port position: pre-port, port, and post-port:

- The skin around the inlet ports must be carefully protected by means of using an adequate port sutured to the skin to avoid the port-site burns.
- Soaked wet drapes especially in the skin close to the proximal end of the probe is useful to prevent the pre-port burns.
- The probe tip can create internal (post-port) burns when it gets too close to the dermis, mainly in two ways: An end hit or a parallel hit. End-hit results when the probe tip is forced injudiciously against the dermis. A parallel-hit

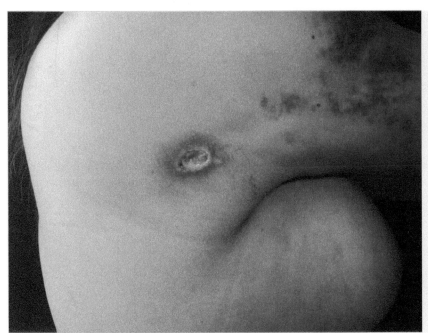

Fig. 11.7 Port burn in the posterior axillary fold and prolonged arm swelling on a 32-year-old female who underwent high definition lipoplasty.

results when the probe lies too superficial and there is either excessive power or insufficient fluid around the probe.

When excessive power is applied and excessive time is used in the deep layer, vascular and fascia injuries may result. This could end up in prolonged bruising, hematoma, abnormal skin retraction, and sensitivity. The way VASER complications can be avoided relies on the correct use and practice of the technique we just explained above. Other complications following VASER technique are derived from the lipoplasty itself and commonly comprise: prolonged edema and bruising, seroma, infections, asymmetries, over-resection, unnatural appearance, bizarre skin retraction and so forth, but they actually overcome the purpose of this chapter. Finally, surgeons must be aware that the proper use of VASER, and other technologies supporting body contour procedures, do require a learning curve and correct training to understand and master their use before trying to improve by our own means.

Suggested Readings

Dalecki D. Mechanical bioeffects of ultrasound. Annu Rev Biomed Eng 2004;6(1):229–248

de Souza Pinto EB, Abdala PC, Maciel CM, dos Santos FdeP, de Souza RPM. Liposuction and VASER. Clin Plast Surg 2006;33(1):107–115, vii

Cimino WW. History of ultrasound-assisted lipoplasty. In: Shiffman MA, Di Giuseppe A, eds. Body contouring: art, science, and clinical practice. Berlin: Springer; 2010:399

Cimino WW. Ultrasonic surgery: power quantification and efficiency optimization. Aesthet Surg J 2001;21(3):233–241

Hoyos AE, Millard JA. VASER-assisted high-definition liposculpture. Aesthet Surg J 2007;27(6):594–604

Jewell ML, Fodor PB, de Souza Pinto EB, Al Shammari MA. Clinical application of VASER-assisted lipoplasty: a pilot clinical study. Aesthet Surg J 2002;22(2):131–146

Miller DL, Smith NB, Bailey MR, Czarnota GJ, Hynynen K, Makin IR; Bioeffects Committee of the American Institute of Ultrasound in Medicine. Overview of therapeutic ultrasound applications and safety considerations. J Ultrasound Med 2012;31(4):623–634

Miller DL, Smith NB, Bailey MR, Czarnota GJ, Hynynen K, Makin IRS, et al. Overview of therapeutic.

Nagy MW, Vanek PF Jr. A multicenter, prospective, randomized, single-blind, controlled clinical trial comparing VASER-assisted Lipoplasty and suction-assisted Lipoplasty. Plast Reconstr Surg 2012;129(4):681e–689e

Ogawa T, Hattori R, Yamamoto T, Gotoh M. Safe use of ultrasonically activated devices based on current studies. Expert Rev Med Devices 2011;8(3):319–324

Panetta NJ, Gupta DM, Kwan MD, Wan DC, Commons GW, Longaker MT. Tissue harvest by means of suction-assisted or third-generation ultrasound-assisted lipoaspiration has no effect on osteogenic potential of human adipose-derived stromal cells. Plast Reconstr Surg 2009;124(1):65–73

Scuderi N, Devita R, D'Andrea F, Vonella M. Nuove prospettive nella liposuzione la lipoemulsica- zone. Giorn Chir Plast Ricostr ed Estetica 1987;2(1):33–39

Schafer ME, Hicok KC, Mills DC, Cohen SR, Chao JJ. Acute adipocyte viability after third-generation ultrasound-assisted liposuction. Aesthet Surg J 2013;33(5):698–704

Zocchi ML. Ultrasonic assisted lipoplasty. Technical refinements and clinical evaluations. Clin Plast Surg 1996;23(4):575–598

12 Water-Assisted Liposuction

Sophie Pei-Hsuan Lu and Steven Hsiang-Ya Wang

Abstract

Water jet-assisted liposuction or water-assisted liposuction (WAL) is one of device-assisted liposuction characterized by water-jet force. WAL offers clinical benefits in decreasing operating time, postoperative swelling, ecchymosis, and pain. The device, operation modes, and techniques of WAL are illustrated in this chapter. In addition, published clinical studies support the high quality of transferrable fat using the LipoCollector system and BEAULI method.

Keywords: Water jet-assisted liposuction, water-assisted liposuction, WAL, body sculpture, BEAULI method, LipoCollector, lipotransfer, fat grafting

---

Key Points

- WAL channels a fan-shaped water jet into adipose tissue to loosen the fatty layer and preserve vital structures.
- The lipoaspirates obtained from WAL can be used for autologous fat transplantation immediately at the same surgical procedure.
- WAL is superior to traditional manual tumescent liposuction in terms of decreasing operating time, postoperative swelling, ecchymosis, and pain.

12.1 Introduction

WAL has been in development since 2000. Inspired by water jet-assisted surgery, WAL is known for preservation of vessels, nerves, and surrounding connective tissue.[1] The German plastic surgeon Ahmed Ziah Taufig was involved in the early development of WAL.[2] The commercial WAL, Body-Jet (Human Med AG, Schwerin, Germany), came to the market in 2004. WAL can be done under local anesthesia, intravenous anesthesia, or general anesthesia. It uses a fan-shaped liquid jet with adjustable pressures to decompose the fat tissue into fragments.[2] The fragmented fat tissue can be suctioned off from the same cannula and then be collected in a lipocollector.[3]

12.2 Patient Selection

The patient selection is as important as any other surgery procedure.

12.2.1 Indications

- Body shaping and liposculpture: face, neck, arms, abdomen, flank, back, hips, brassiere rolls, lumbar rolls, banana rolls, axillary rolls, thighs, calves, etc.[4]
- Gynecomastia.[5]
- Combined procedures with fat grafting to the face, breasts, buttock, etc.[6]

12.2.2 Contraindications

- Heavy smoker.
- Diabetes mellitus without control.

- Severe coagulation disorders.
- Unrealistic expectations.

12.3 Technique

WAL incorporates a dual-chambered cannula that simultaneously emits fan-shaped jets of tumescent solution and removes fatty tissue with the infiltrated subcutaneous fluid. The advantage of water-jet dissection is the preservation of vessels and nerves. According to one study on the abdominal fat tissue of fresh cadavers, the optimal pressure for water-jet dissection of fatty tissue lies between 30 and 40 Bar.[1]

12.3.1 Device

Functional Elements (▶Fig. 12.1)

- **Rack with hooks and weighing system** is used to hold the fluid bags. Each hook carries one fluid bag.
- **Swivel lever** is used to fold the rack down for transportation.
- **Touch screen** is used for operating the device.
- **Suction container** includes suction bags with angle connector. There are two identical suction containers on the Body-Jet to house the disposable suction bags.

These are inserted into the suction containers and are used for collection of the excessive aspirate.

Control Panel for Device Operation (▶Fig. 12.2)

- **Touch-screen** is used for operating the device.
- **Display of the operational state of the device.**
- **'Stop' key** is used for immediate deactivation of the water, jet generation, and the suctioning in case of hazardous or error situations.
- **Keys for selection of the suction container.**

Cannulas

Infiltration Cannulas (▶Fig. 12.3)

Infiltration cannulas are used to preinfiltrate the suction area with tumescent solution for anesthesia and vasoconstriction. They have no side holes in order to avoid reflux of fluid. The spray-jet is pointing upwards.

Standard WAL Cannulas (▶Fig. 12.4)

Standard WAL cannulas come in four diameters (3.5 mm, 3.8 mm, 4.2 mm, 4.8 mm) and three lengths (15 cm, 25 cm, 30 cm). They have four suction holes. The spray-jet is pointing upwards.

Rapid WAL Cannulas (▶Fig. 12.5)

Rapid WAL cannulas are available in two diameters (3.5 mm, 3.8 mm) and three lengths (15 cm, 25 cm, 30 cm). They have four suction holes with a sharpened edge geometry, which facilitates suction in scarred or fibrous areas. The spray-jet is pointing upwards.

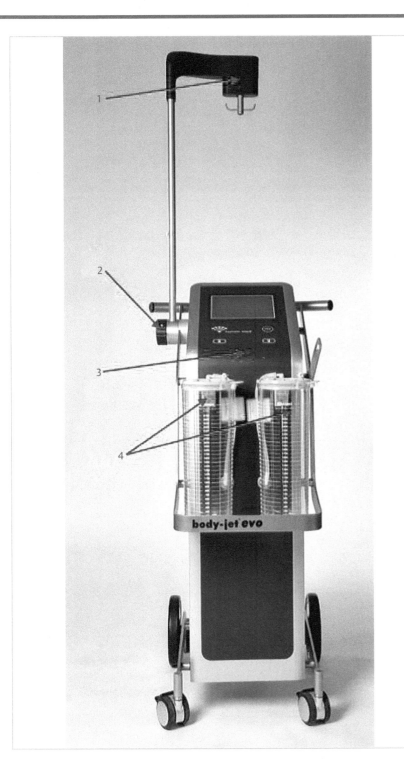

Fig. 12.1 Functional elements of the water jet-assisted liposuction device. **(1)** Rack with hooks and weighing system is used to hold the fluid bags. Each hook carries one fluid bag. **(2)** Swivel lever is used to fold the rack down for transportation. **(3)** Touch screen is used for operating the device. **(4)** Suction container includes suction bags with angle connector. There are two identical suction containers on the Body-Jet to house the disposable suction bags. These are inserted into the suction containers and are used for collection of the excessive aspirate.

Subcutaneous WAL Cannulas (▶Fig. 12.6)

Subcutaneous WAL cannulas are used in very superficial and sensitive areas based on the design of the suction holes and spray-jet pointing downwards. This keeps spray and suction away from skin or fascia. They come in two diameters (3.5 mm, 3.8 mm), two lengths (25 cm, 30 cm), and two hole configurations (two or three suction holes).

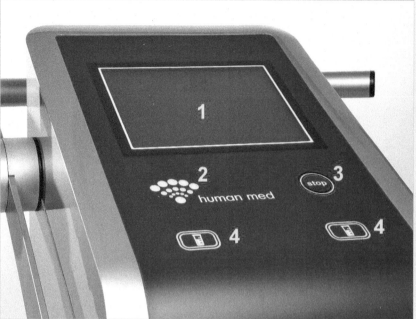

Fig. 12.2 Control panel for device operation **(1)** Touch-screen is used for operating the device. **(2)** Display of the operational state of the device. **(3)** 'Stop' key is used for immediate deactivation of the water, jet generation and the suctioning in case of hazardous or error situations. **(4)** Keys for selection of the suction container.

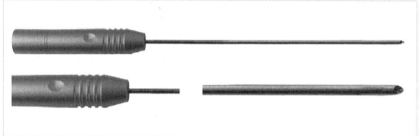

Fig. 12.3 Infiltration WAL cannulas. Infiltration cannulas are used to pre-infiltrate the suction area with tumescent solution for anesthesia and vasoconstriction. They have no side holes in order to avoid reflux of fluid. The spray-jet is pointing upwards.

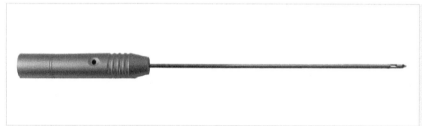

Fig. 12.4 Standard WAL cannulas. Standard WAL cannulas come in four diameters (3.5 mm, 3.8 mm, 4.2 mm, 4.8 mm) and three lengths (15 cm, 25 cm, 30 cm). They have four suction holes. The spray-jet is pointing upwards.

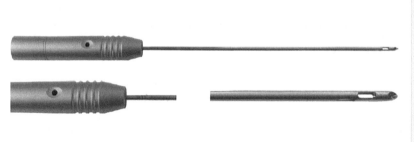

Fig. 12.5 Rapid WAL cannulas. Rapid WAL cannulas are available in two diameters (3.5 mm, 3.8 mm) and three lengths (15 cm, 25 cm, 30 cm). They have four suction holes with a sharpened edge geometry, which facilitates suction in scarred or fibrous areas. The spray-jet is pointing upwards.

12.3.2 WAL Operating Modes (▶Fig. 12.7)

Short Mode

- Even and low pain induction with good subdermal infiltration.
- Very easy working and guiding of the cannula, especially in fibrotic tissue.

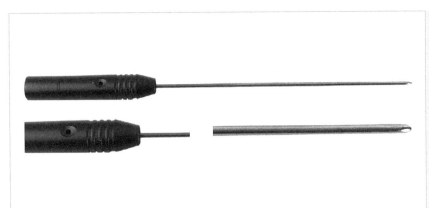

Fig. 12.6 Subcutaneous WAL cannulas. Subcutaneous WAL cannulas are used in very superficial and sensitive area based on the design of the suction holes and spray-jet pointing downwards. This keeps spray and suction away from skin or fascia. They come in two diameters (3.5 mm, 3.8 mm), two lengths (25 cm, 30 cm) and two hole configurations (two or three suction holes).

The flow rate of each pulsation mode and range

	Pulsation mode		
	Short	Medium	Long
Range		Flow rate in ml/min	
1	100	92	152
2	116	116	164
3	132	128	176
4	148	148	188

The water jet pressure of each pulsation mode and range

	Pulsation mode		
	Short	Medium	Long
Range		Pressure in bar	
1	30	30	30
2	40	50	40
3	50	70	50
4	70	90	70

Fig. 12.7 The flow rate of each pulsation mode and range of the Body-Jet. The surgeons can choose appropriate flow rate and pressure for each area of water-assisted liposuction.

• Fast and smooth-running of fat harvesting.
• Most effective for gentle liposuction and body contouring and fat harvesting.
• Easy learning curve.

Medium Mode

• The prototype water-jet mode of the first Body-Jet generation.
• Scientifically proven clinical results.

Long Mode

• Optimum mode for cell saving and effective harvesting of vital fat tissue including viable stromal vascular fraction/stem cells.
• Long spray intervals with short interruptions.
• Fast and time-saving infiltration of larger volumes of tumescent, especially in deep layer.
• Designed for quick tissue expansion.

12.3.3 Sequences

The sequences of WAL can be divided as follows.

Phase 1: Infiltration

For Liposculpture

• Mode: Short/medium.
• Range: 1–2.
• 100 mL of tumescent for a palm-sized area.
• Stay for 7–10 minutes.

For Fat Harvesting

• Mode: Long.
• Range: 12.
• 100 mL of tumescent for a palm sized area.
• Stay for 35 minutes.

Phase 2: Simultaneous Infiltration and Aspiration

Phase 3: Drying or Finishing

A variable-force infusion pump drives the infiltration solution through a closed tubing system into a passageway within the application cannula.[6] The fluid streams out from the cannulas nozzle tip at a 30° angle to loosen the fatty tissue. The washed-out fatty tissue is evacuated from surgical sites through a separate channel within the cannula, which is connected to an integrated suction unit. The application cannulas vary in diameter, arrangement, and sharpness of openings. The flow rate of the infiltrate, as well as the application of variable intensities of negative pressure, can be selected at different levels, depending on the purpose. A sterile container can be connected between the working cannula and the suction pump to collect the aspirate under reduced negative pressures. The fat is separated from the infranate for immediate usage without centrifugation. WAL relies on two tumescent subcutaneous infiltration solutions. A higher concentration of lidocaine in the infiltration solution is employed during Phase 1 to provide longer-lasting local anesthesia and vasoconstriction. A solution with lower lidocaine concentration is instilled during Phase 2 (simultaneous infiltration and aspiration), along with Phase 3 (drying or finishing) to reduce the pharmacological effects of lidocaine and the accompanying fluid load.

12.3.4 Tumescent Solution

The tumescent solution (▶ Fig. 12.8) suggested in the use of WAL is described as the Berlin Autologous Lipotransfer (BEAULI Method).[3] The BEAULI Method refers to autologous fat grafts collected with the Body-Jet by WAL.

12.3.5 LipoCollector

The aspirated fat particles can be continuously transported to the sterile closed collecting system (LipoCollector, human med AG, Schwerin, Germany).

In the LipoCollector (▶ Fig. 12.9), unwanted fibrous structures and liquids are filtered and mostly eliminated. The collected fat particles can be used for grafting immediately under the circumstances that the exposure of the fat to oxygen or contaminants is reduced to a minimum.

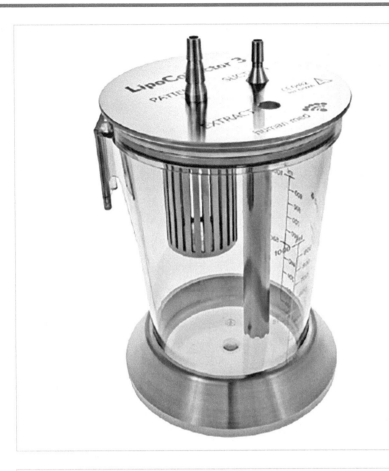

Fig. 12.8 The tumescent method to WAL technique: the BEAULI Method. Phase 1 is infiltration of tumescent. Phase 2 is simultaneous infiltration of tumescent and aspiration of fat.

Fig. 12.9 The LipoCollector of the Body-Jet system. The sterile LipoCollector enables immediate lipotransfer after water-assisted liposuction.

The tumescent method to WAL technique
<the Beauli Method>

	Phase 1	Phase 2
Xylocaine 1% (10 mg/ml)	50 ml	25 ml
Suprarenin 1:1,000 (Epinephrin)	1 ml	1 ml
Sodium bicarbonate 8.4% (NaHCO₃)	20 ml	20 ml

Per 1,000 ml NaCl (0.9%)
Warm to 35°C, cooling of fat and prevent body chilling

12.3.6 Aftercare

The aftercare in WAL is the same as in other liposuction procedures. There will be slight swelling and pain within the first 2 to 3 days after the WAL. The bruises will disappear after 2 to 4 weeks. The suture stiches are removed after 5 to 7 days. The compression garment use is recommended as the following protocol:

• Wear compression garment immediately after surgery and for at least one month.
• Within 1–2 weeks after surgery, it must be worn every day for 24 hours a day.
• Within 3–4 weeks after surgery, it must be worn every day for 12 hours a day or more (subject to availability).

Initial results may be immediately noticeable and effects will be more apparent after 3 to 7 days. Postoperative massage can be started 2 weeks after surgery to promote skin retraction.

12.4 Clinical Applications

- Thigh liposuction (▶Fig. 12.10a, b)
- Arm liposuction (▶Fig. 12.11a, b)
- Abdomen liposuction (▶Fig. 12.12a, b)
- Breast lipofilling (▶Fig. 12.13 a, b)

The fat particles collected by the WAL can be immediately reinjected into the recipient area with or without further surgical procedures.

12.5 Combination Treatment

A recent randomized controlled study comparing lipoaspirates obtaining from WAL and conventional manual liposuction revealed greater viability, better weight retention, less apoptosis, and greater angiogenesis in the WAL group.[7] Preliminary experiences on 132 patients (240 breasts) undergoing 487 autologous water jet-assisted fat grafting procedures reported minor complications (5.35%), like tiny oil cysts formation and hematoma of the donor site.[8]

12.5.1 Autologous Fat Transplantation

Before the Breast Autologous Fat Transplantation (AFT)

- Breast physical examination.
- No over-expectation: one cup increase in the breast size in a session.
- Mammography if more than 40 years of age.
- Routine breast echo exam and documentation.
- Informed consent: cyst, calcification, fat necrosis, but unlikely increase cancer risk according to the record to date.

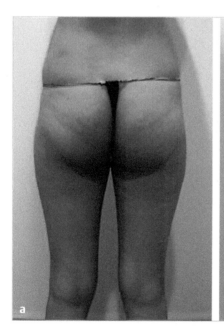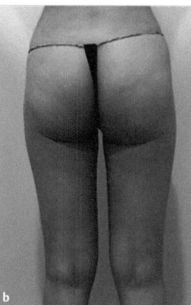

Fig. 12.10 (**a, b**) Before and after photos of circumferential thigh liposuction by water-assisted liposuction.

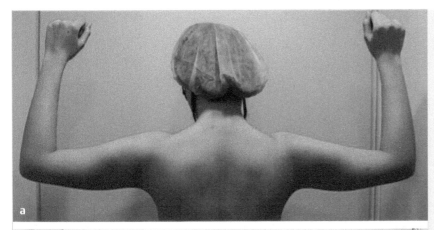

Fig. 12.11 (**a, b**) Before and after photos of arm liposuction by water-assisted liposuction.

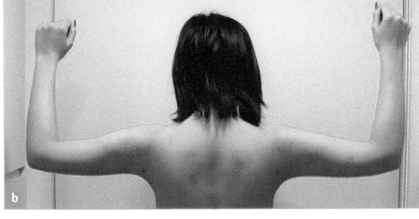

Fig. 12.12 (**a, b**) Before and after photos of circumferential abdomen liposuction by water-assisted liposuction.

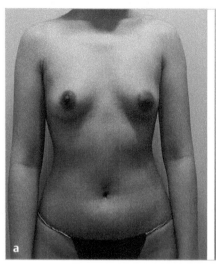 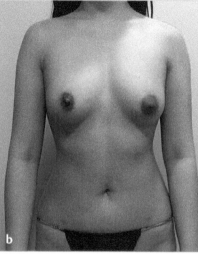

Fig. 12.13 (a, b) Before and after photos of circumferential abdomen liposuction and fat transfer to the breast area. The fat particles collected by the LipoCollector can be immediately reinjected into the recipient area.

• Measure for elasticity.
• Preoperative markings on donor sites and breasts as cosmetic subunits.

BEAULI Method for Fat Harvesting and Grafting

Step 1: Collecting and Rinsing of Fat Tissue

• Decant: 20 to 30 minutes is long enough to separate the blood and the tumescent solution.

Step 2: Preparing for AFT (for Direct Injection)

• 10 mL syringe for breast AFT.
• 1 or 3 mL BD syringe for fat grafting on face or hands.
• 18 gauge dull tip cannula for grafting.

12.6 Pros and Cons of the WAL

12.6.1 Pros

Operating Time

• Less operating time in WAL compared to traditional liposuction; theoretically decreasing the risks associated with anesthesia and the incidence of pulmonary embolism.[9]

Time of Tumescent Solution Remaining in the Tissue

• Less time of tumescent solution remaining in the tissue in WAL compared to traditional tumescent liposuction, less intraoperative swelling allows for more precise determination of the target result, and decreased postoperative swelling.[6]

Postoperative Pain

• Less postoperative pain in WAL compared to traditional liposuction.[9]

Postoperative Ecchymosis

• Less postoperative ecchymosis in WAL compared to traditional liposuction.[9]

12.6.2 Cons

Learning Curve

• Learning time required for surgeons.[6]

12.6.3 Device and Disposables

• Device and disposables required for practice.

References

[1] Wanner M, Jakob S, Schwarzl E, Oberholzer M, Pierer G. Optimizing the parameters for hydro-jet dissection in fatty tissue: a morphological ex vivo analysis. Eur Surg 2002;34(2):134–142

[2] Taufig AZ. Water-jet assisted liposucion. In: Liposuction: principles and practice. Springer; 2006; 326–330

[3] Ueberreiter K, Tanzella U, Cromme F, Doll D, Krapohl BD. One stage rescue procedure after capsular contracture of breast implants with autologous fat grafts collected by water assisted liposuction ("BEAULI Method"). GMS Interdisciplinary Plastic and Reconstructive Surgery DGPW 2013, Vol. 2, ISSN 2193–8091

[4] Sasaki GH. Water-assisted liposuction for body contouring and lipoharvesting: safety and efficacy in 41 consecutive patients. Aesthet Surg J 2011;31(1):76–88

[5] Wolter A, Scholz T, Diedrichson J, Liebau J. [Surgical treaent of gynecomastia: an algorithm] Handchir Mikrochir Plast Chir 2013;45(2):73–79

[6] Man D, Meyer H. Water jet-assisted lipoplasty. Aesthet Surg J 2007;27(3):342–346

[7] Yin S, Luan J, Fu S, Wang Q, Zhuang Q. Does water-jet force make a difference in fat grafting? In vitro and in vivo evidence of improved lipoaspirate viability and fat graft survival. Plast Reconstr Surg 2015;135(1):127–138

[8] Stabile M, Ueberreiter K, Schaller HE, Hoppe DL. Jet-assisted fat transfer to the female breast: preliminary experiences. Eur J Plast Surg 2014;37(5):267–272

[9] Araco A, Gravante G, Araco F, Delogu D, Cervelli V. Comparison of power water–assisted and traditional liposuction: a prospective randomized trial of postoperative pain. Aesthetic Plast Surg 2007;31(3):259–265

13 Power-Assisted Liposuction Cannula Types and Technique

Briar L. Dent and B. Aviva Preminger

Abstract

Power-assisted liposuction (PAL) allows for increased fat extraction with reduced tissue trauma and operator fatigue due to improved tissue penetration. The reciprocating motion and device vibration facilitate more rapid fat aspiration with decreased physical exertion particularly in fibrous areas and revision procedures. Studies have demonstrated larger volume fat aspiration and shorter operative times and potential skin tightening. Additional benefits reported include less intraoperative and postoperative pain, less postoperative ecchymosis and edema and greater patient satisfaction when compared to traditional liposuction techniques. The reduced adipocyte damage may also allow for improved fat grafting. PAL has, therefore, become a proven technique with advantages over traditional liposuction.

Keywords: Power-assisted liposuction, liposuction, fat grafting, gynecomastia, fat harvest, energy-assisted liposuction, fat aspiration

> *"Nearly all men can stand adversity, but if you want to test a man's character, give him power."*
>
> —Abraham Lincoln

13.1 History of PAL

Liposuction as a procedure has always been a balance between the need to maximize tissue penetration and minimize tissue damage. PAL was developed in the 1990s in response to the need for improved fat penetration and control without the generation of excessive heat and the complications associated with ultrasound-based devices.[1]

13.2 Equipment

The first power-assisted devices incorporated a blade within a cannula drawing from orthopedic and otolaryngologic instruments and were primarily intended for submental use.[2] Concerns about increased blood loss using cannulas with internal blades led manufacturers away from blades in favor of reciprocating cannulas.[2] These instruments were designed to vibrate at a rate of 800 to 10,000 movements per minute and the vibration allowed easier tissue penetration.[2] The power-assisted devices were also designed to work with a variety of cannula shapes and sizes.

The early powered devices were driven by compressed gas and were very noisy.[2,3] They also required the expense and inconvenience of maintaining large tanks of medical-grade compressed gas. Byron Surgical (Mentor, Irvine CA) developed a disposable power-assisted handle that was driven by the air discharged from the aspirator.[2] However, this was fraught with increased noise and cost. Quieter electrical sources were soon developed.[3]

A small variable speed motor generates a forward and backward reciprocating motion to produce a 2 mm to 12 mm excursion at the tip.[4,5,6] At the tissue level, the reciprocating movements of the powered cannula mirror that of the manual movements but the standard stroke distance and limited lateral movements help to reduce tissue trauma. Vigorous movements are replaced by slower manual passes of the powered cannula, maximizing fat extraction with less exertion. The mechanism of action has not been clearly defined. Two possibilities have been proposed: (1) a jackhammer-type motion of the cannula tip breaks up fat or (2) the fat is suctioned into the cannula and then avulsed by the reciprocating motion.[4]

Studies have demonstrated the largest increase in fat extraction using the PAL system previously produced by Byron Surgical (Mentor, Irvine CA).[2] Some systems rely on electricity and others are gas driven.[6] Differences in efficacy may be attributable to differences in the rate of vibration though it is unclear whether slower or faster vibration provides optimal efficiency for removing fat.[2] The extent of radial movement may also contribute to efficacy. Choice among competing PAL devices is generally based upon warrantee, preference of electrical versus pneumatic, vibration, and noise.[6] In the United States, the PAL LipoSculptor by MicroAire (Charlottesville, VA) is the only PAL system that is currently being manufactured. The device is electric and operates with a 2 mm reciprocating stroke at 4,000 cycles per minute. Per report from the manufacturer in 2016, the system costs approximately US$20,000. Other companies that have previously manufactured PAL systems include Wells-Johnson (Tucson AZ), Byron Surgical (Mentor, Irvine CA), and Medtronic (Minneapolis MN), but these products are no longer on the market.

Powered systems incorporate cannulas of comparable length and diameter to suction-assisted lipoplasty cannulas, allowing for the use of small incisions. The powered cannulas have been shown to create larger tunnels in the subcutaneous tissue than traditional liposuction cannulas.[2,7] In other words, a 3 mm cannula may produce tunnels of 4 mm or larger.[2,7] Therefore, surgeons should consider choosing a smaller size cannula than that to which they are usually accustomed. This also allows surgeons to make smaller access incisions than they would typically require for a given tunnel size. When the power is on, the cannula can be held in one place and still remove fat. Caution must be used for this same reason to avoid creating contour irregularities.

13.3 Advantages for the Surgeon

The improved tissue penetration of the power-assisted devices reduces operator fatigue by allowing for more rapid aspiration and decreased muscle strain. This is particularly helpful in revision cases as well as fibrous areas such as the back, flanks, and male breast. By reducing the physical exertion required by the surgeon, longer or more numerous surgeries can potentially be performed in a given session. Furthermore, decreasing the fatigue and monotony associated with traditional liposuction likely improves surgeon attention and precision.[2,7,8]

A multicenter study performed by Coleman et al demonstrated an average increase in fat extraction of 30% (range 20 to 45%) with PAL, as compared to traditional liposuction.[5] Traditional liposuction was simulated in their study by using PAL devices in their non-powered modes. The greatest increase in fat extraction was seen in the hip area (62%), compared to the upper thighs (48%) and the abdomen (36%), which supports the observation that PAL is particularly advantageous in fibrous areas where traditional liposuction can be more challenging.

Katz et al compared traditional liposuction and PAL in a group of patients who served as their own controls.[7] They found that PAL was associated with 35% shorter operative times, 31% greater fat aspiration per minute, and 49% less surgeon fatigue than traditional liposuction.[7] The authors also reported that, because of the greater ease with which the powered cannula moves within the subcutaneous tissue, together with the increased patient comfort associated with PAL (see section 13.4), they were able to fine-tune difficult areas at the end of the case with the patient standing.[2,7] They believe that this opportunity allows for a degree of final symmetry and contour that could not otherwise be achieved with traditional liposuction and a lower incidence of revision procedures.[7]

In an attempt to assess skin tightening following PAL, Sasaki et al measured surface area changes in three patients who underwent both PAL and traditional liposuction of their abdomen.[9] While their results did not reach statistical significance, they reported a greater reduction in skin surface area with PAL (average 5.8%) than with traditional liposuction (average 4.2%) six months postoperatively.[9] Their study was limited by its small sample size, but should encourage further research into the potential skin tightening advantages of PAL over traditional liposuction.

The overall increase in fat extraction reported by Coleman et al, as discussed above, was only significant for surgeons who had performed eight or more PAL cases.[5] For surgeons who had performed seven or fewer PAL cases, there was no significant difference in fat extraction between powered and non-powered liposuction. The study draws attention to the short but real learning curve associated with the powered devices. Surgeons must become accustomed to moving the cannula more slowly than in traditional liposuction in order to maximize the fat extraction benefits of PAL. While temporary, this learning curve may be considered a small disadvantage of PAL.

13.4 Advantages for the Patient

Since power-assisted devices improve the tissue penetration associated with each cannula stroke, the process is less traumatic to the patient's tissue than traditional liposuction for a given volume of aspirate. This reduces tissue trauma, edema, and ecchymosis, and thereby reduces recovery time for the patient.[1,8] Unlike ultrasound-assisted liposuction, which also offers the advantage of improved tissue penetration, PAL does not carry the associated risk of thermal injury.[8] The vibration produced by the power-assisted device is also believed to create a distracting neuronal sensation that helps to decrease the perception of pain.[2,5,6,7] Many patients prefer this vibration to the jabbing or tearing sensation associated with traditional liposuction.[2,5,6,7] All of the above factors allow PAL to be easily performed under local anesthesia, which is often more convenient, safer, and less expensive for the patient than general anesthesia.

Katz et al found that PAL was associated with 45% less intraoperative pain, 35 to 38% less postoperative pain, 37 to 48% less postoperative ecchymosis, 27 to 32% less postoperative edema, and greater patient satisfaction with results when compared to traditional liposuction.[7] Similarly, Coleman et al found that 54% of the patients in their multicenter study preferred PAL to traditional liposuction, 46% had no preference, and none preferred traditional liposuction.[5]

13.5 Procedure

Preoperative photographs are taken, and the patient is marked in the standing position. Incision sites can be designed asymmetrically to help reduce the stigmata of liposuction.[2] Tumescent anesthesia is infiltrated and allowed at least 15 minutes for full vasoconstrictive effect prior to commencing suctioning. The powered cannula is assembled and connected to the aspiration hose. The number of strokes per minute is preset on the power console depending on the brand and ranges from 800 to 10,000.[2]

Once the desired result has been obtained with the patient in a recumbent or lateral decubitus position, Katz et al advocate re-assessing the patient in a standing position in order to perform any necessary touch-ups prior to completion of the operation.[2] This allows the surgeon an opportunity to assess contours that may have changed with gravity or compression while the patient was lying down. If the operating room is equipped with a camera and television monitor, the patient can also review images and give additional feedback.

Postoperatively, patients are instructed to wear a moderate compression garment to facilitate lymphatic return and decrease seroma formation.

13.6 Complications

Compared to traditional liposuction cannulas, more local tissue damage could theoretically occur if a power-assisted cannula was left in one place for a prolonged interval since the cannula will continue to extract fat, even when stationary. We have not, however, found any reports of this problem in the literature.

In theory, the complication profile associated with PAL should parallel that of traditional liposuction and we should expect to see patients with seromas and contour irregularities, as well as rare cases of infection, hypotension, hemorrhage, shock, anesthetic toxicity, cardiac arrhythmia, nerve damage, violation of the abdominal or thoracic wall with viscus perforation, pulmonary thromboembolism, fat embolism, and death. Due perhaps to the relatively recent adoption of this technology, not all of these complications have been reported in the literature.

A study by Katz et al of complications following PAL reported an overall complication rate of 1.4%, which is comparable to that of traditional liposuction performed with tumescent anesthesia.[8] This corresponded to 3 postoperative seromas in a group of 207 patients, all of which were successfully treated with aspiration and compression. They did not report any systemic complications.

In a study of 547 PAL cases by Sasaki et al, complications included fibrotic nodule formation (5%), prolonged induration (3%), and seroma (less than 1%).[9] The fibrotic nodules all resolved spontaneously or following intralesional steroid injection and ultrasound therapy. The seromas all resolved spontaneously without aspiration. They did not experience any systemic complications.

13.7 New Applications

Since PAL allows for more efficient fat extraction than traditional liposuction, causes less adipocyte damage than ultrasound-based devices, and facilitates suctioning of fibrous areas, it has the potential to be very useful in fat grafting and liposculpture. Keck et al compared samples of abdominal fat harvested by PAL and traditional liposuction and reported comparable numbers of viable adipose-derived stem cells and cellular proliferation rates between the groups in vitro.[10] Interestingly, the cells harvested using PAL showed significantly higher expression levels of differentiation markers adiponectin, GLUT4, and PPAR, which promote the differentiation of stem cells into mature adipocytes, than the cells harvested using traditional liposuction. Codazzi et al reported successful clinical results using a PAL device to harvest fat for fat grafting and liposculpture.[11]

Abboud et al describe a combination of PAL and subsequent fat transfer for the treatment of mild to moderate brachial ptosis that obviates the need for skin excision.[12] They perform PAL of the posterior arm and para-axillary region, followed by lipofilling of the bicipital triangle of the medial upper arm, which they believe restores an aesthetically pleasing contour and helps to lift the ptotic skin of the posterior arm. They report 90% patient satisfaction. The authors feel that this procedure offers an effective alternative to traditional brachioplasty with skin excision that is associated with shorter operative times, faster patient recovery, minimal scarring, and fewer postoperative complications.

Multiple studies have reported successful results using PAL in the treatment of gynecomastia.[13,14] Since PAL is particularly effective at suctioning fibrous areas, it is better suited than traditional liposuction for contouring the dense fat and fibroglandular tissue of the male breast. Lista et al report excellent results using PAL and a subsequent pull-through technique in a study of 99 patients (197 breasts) with gynecomastia.[13] Only 3 of 99 patients (5 breasts) required an additional peri-areolar incision to remove residual breast tissue. For the 96 successful cases, a single 4 mm access incision was made at the lateral aspect of the inframammary fold and an average of 459 mL of lipoaspirate was removed, followed by 5 to 70 grams of resected tissue. None of the patients required a revision surgery. The authors believe that this technique consistently produces a naturally contoured male breast. Similarly, Scuderi et al describe the use of PAL with a transareolar incision for the treatment of mild to moderate gynecomastia.[14] They recommend the use of two small liposuction access sites at the lateral inframammary fold and axillary origin. If a residual mound of breast tissue remains beneath the nipple and areola after completion of PAL, they perform a transareolar incision to directly excise this tissue. In their study of 23 patients, lipoaspirate volume ranged from 100 to 400 mL and parenchymal excision from 20 to 110 grams.

13.8 Conclusion

Since its development in the 1990s, PAL has become a useful technique with many advantages over traditional liposuction for the surgeon and patient alike. For the surgeon, PAL provides greater tissue penetration with increased fat extraction, facilitates suctioning of fibrous areas, decreases operator fatigue, and shortens operative times. For the patient, PAL offers reduced intraoperative and postoperative pain, less postoperative edema and ecchymosis, and potentially greater overall satisfaction. Disadvantages of the technique consist mainly of a small learning curve, increased noise, and the expense of purchasing the equipment. In addition to its use in routine liposuction, PAL has shown promising results in fat grafting and liposculpture, body contouring, and the treatment of gynecomastia.

References

[1] Rebelo A. Power-assisted liposuction. Clin Plast Surg 2006; 33(1):91–105, vii

[2] Katz BE, Maiwald DC. Power liposuction. Dermatol Clin 2005; 23(3):383–391, v

[3] Shridharani SM, Broyles JM, Matarasso A. Liposuction devices: technology update. Med Devices (Auckl) 2014; 7:241–251

[4] Young VL; Plastic Surgery Educational Foundation DATA Committee. Power-assisted lipoplasty. Plast Reconstr Surg 2001; 108(5):1429–1432

[5] Coleman WP, III, Katz B, Bruck M, et al. The efficacy of powered liposuction. Dermatol Surg 2001; 27(8):735–738

[6] Flynn TC. Powered liposuction: an evaluation of currently available instrumentation. Dermatol Surg 2002; 28(5):376–382

[7] Katz BE, Bruck MC, Coleman WP, III. The benefits of powered liposuction versus traditional liposuction: a paired comparison analysis. Dermatol Surg 2001; 27(10):863–867

[8] Katz BE, Bruck MC, Felsenfeld L, Frew KE. Power liposuction: a report on complications. Dermatol Surg 2003; 29(9):925–927, discussion 927

[9] Sasaki GH, Tevez A, Ulloa EL. Power-assisted liposuction (PAL) vs. traditional liposuction: quantification and comparison of tissue shrinkage and tightening. In: Serdev N, ed. Advanced techniques in liposuction and fat transfer. Intech; 2011

[10] Keck M, Kober J, Riedl O, et al. Power assisted liposuction to obtain adipose-derived stem cells: impact on viability and differentiation to adipocytes in comparison to manual aspiration. J Plast Reconstr Aesthet Surg 2014; 67(1):e1–e8

[11] Codazzi D, Bruschi S, Robotti E, Bocchiotti MA. Power-assisted liposuction (P.A.L.) fat harvesting for lipofilling: the trap device. World J Plast Surg 2015; 4(2):177–179

[12] Abboud MH, Abboud NM, Dibo SA. Brachioplasty by power-assisted liposuction and fat transfer: a novel approach that obviates skin excision. Aesthet Surg J 2016; 36(8):908–917

[13] Lista F, Ahmad J. Power-assisted liposuction and the pull-through technique for the treatment of gynecomastia. Plast Reconstr Surg 2008; 121(3):740–747

[14] Scuderi N, Dessy LA, Tempesta M, Bistoni G, Mazzocchi M. Combined use of power-assisted liposuction and trans-areolar incision for gynaecomastia treatment. J Plast Reconstr Aesthet Surg 2010; 63(1):e93–e95

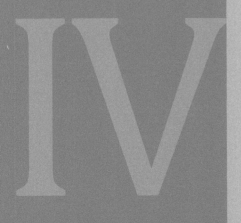

Section IV

Technology-Based Body Contouring by Anatomy

IV

14 Scarless Face Lifting with Bipolar Radiofrequency Assistance

Diane Irvine Duncan

Abstract

Traditional face lifting techniques have been replaced in a majority of patients with a multitude of less invasive options, including botulinum toxin and filler injections, fat transfer, laser resurfacing, transcutaneous MFU and RF, and needling techniques. While these approaches certainly help deter the appearance of aging, neither surgical face lifting nor the aforementioned options address the root cause of facial skin laxity. As people age, a structural change in the adipose layer creates apparent skin laxity. The adipose framework that the skin rests upon loses the integrity of its collagen structure over years. In a manner similar to the well-known atrophy of facial fat, the stroma/vascular fraction also undergoes erosion. Clinical manifestations of this process include the descent of facial fullness downwards towards the nasolabial folds and jowls. Correction of the process includes the restoration of a three dimensional framework in the superficial adipose layer. Utilization of bipolar radiofrequency (RF) in the subcutaneous layer of the neck and midface can restore the fine fibrous network that supports the facial shape. The results improve with time up to one year. The procedure can safely be combined with other approaches in order to optimize outcome. Because the root cause of skin and soft tissue laxity is corrected, the longevity of results with this method of treatment surpasses that of traditional surgical techniques.

Keywords: Radiofrequency, skin tightening, midface lifting, nonexcisional, regenerative, minimal downtime

---

Key Points

- Technique used for patients with mild to moderate facial laxity.
- Addresses root cause of soft tissue laxity.
- Results improve with time over one year.
- Lift is limited to about 30% contraction of the skin envelope.
- Support garment should be used in order to enhance outcome.
- Results vary; not all patients respond in a similar manner.
- Central facial problems not effectively addressed with traditional face lifting techniques can be addressed well without skin excision.

14.1 Introduction

In 2010, a small version of a bipolar radiofrequency device became available under IRB oversight for treatment of face and neck for skin and soft tissue laxity. At that time, the lack of a stromal collagen support matrix was not recognized as a root cause of apparent facial aging. Therefore, the development of this scarless facelift took several years. Initially, the device was used to augment treatment of focal laxity in conjunction with an open facelift. Those regions treated were regions known to be poorly corrected with traditional excisional techniques. The nasolabial fold, marionette lines, central submental, and jowl regions were initially targeted.

Patients were treated with the bipolar radiofrequency-based device over a five year period. The simple procedure included infusion of tumescent fluid followed by bipolar RF minimally invasive soft tissue tightening for a variety of indications. The majority of patients underwent radiofrequency-assisted treatment for the purpose of aiding an open or short scar facelift approach. This approach was also used for secondary facelifts, as central residual or recurrent laxity was noted frequently as a chief complaint.

14.2 Indications: Choosing a Patient

The ideal patient meets the following criteria:
- Desires mild to moderate face lifting without the scars associated with a traditional skin excision technique.
- The procedure can be used in both men and women.
- Patients with limited recovery time may choose this technique as downtime is usually 2–3 days. Mild bruising and swelling may occur. Patients may return to work whenever the degree of swelling is acceptable, and residual bruising can be covered with makeup.
- Compliance with wearing a support garment for 2–3 days initially, and for 2 weeks postoperatively at night will improve the outcome. In difficult cases combining a heavy face/neck with liposuction, or a secondary correction, the face and neck compression garment worn at night for a longer period can help mold the face and reduce contour irregularities. Removing stretch or tension at the treatment site improves the formation of collagen-binding of the tissue matrix over time.
- Willingness to wait for improvement is also necessary; while significant improvement is noted at six weeks post-treatment, the optimal outcome may not be seen for 6–12 months.
- The desire for avoidance of scars must be strong as improvement may be mild to moderate only.

14.3 Contraindications

- Pregnant or nursing patients.
- Patients with unrealistic expectations.
- Unwillingness to comply with wearing of support garments or prolonged follow-up.
- Severe facial skin laxity, or severe soft tissue laxity.
- The presence of very thick skin, scars, or fibrosis from previous surgeries.
- Obese patients.

14.4 Technique

Technique with this approach starts with good patient selection. If the problem you are hoping to correct is small enough to be effectively addressed with this procedure, then it can be considered. In first evaluating the patient, it is important to have an understanding of how much this procedure can accomplish. Localized bulges can be flattened, and some degree of focal skin ptosis and laxity can be improved. Predictability of outcome is a learned skill; it is best to start small when first attempting this procedure.

Tumescent fluid is infused as it would be for liposuction. Because the facial nerves could be at risk, more infusion is generally safer than just a little. Depending upon the area to be treated, I will inject 100–200 cc of standard tumescent solution per facial side, superficially, after marking the target regions in an upright position. The well-known trouble spots where the facial nerve becomes superficial are marked before tumescing, as these can become distorted after infusing. However, generally no liposuction is used. I prefer bipolar radiofrequency minimally invasive devices for this procedure, but monopolar RF can also be used. The external temperature is not allowed to exceed 35 degrees Centigrade. My maximum internal temperature is 55 degrees. Keeping settings safe ensures that adequate time on tissue can be achieved without damaging facial nerves or creating a burn. It is important to respect the small amount of tissue you are working with.

For best results, the entire skin envelope that has subcutaneous fat below it is treated ▶ Fig. 14.1. I avoid the forehead as heating the frontalis muscle is not very effective and can be quite risky. Energy used can vary from 1–4 kilojoules per side, depending on the location and severity of the problem being treated. Especially for beginners, I would not recommend overtreatment. A flattened look will not be attractive. Overtreatment can cause a focal depression which can be irreversible.

Clinical endpoints include an audible crackling of tumesced tissue combined with a visible tissue response. In most regions, this will be a slight flattening of the protuberant area. Another visible change can be the erasure of fine lines or crepiness. Tissue will heat up quickly so if the maximum temperatures have been reached, move elsewhere. If the problem is severe and you are strongly inclined to retreat the same area, it is a good idea to let the soft tissue temperature return to normal before beginning a brief second session.

Access ports are usually made with an 18 gauge Nocor type needle, which is often used for subcision. A standard 18 gauge needle can be used as well. Because these needle pokes are usually very difficult to see, the placement of access ports should be performed with an eye for the clinical effect, not for the purpose of camouflage.

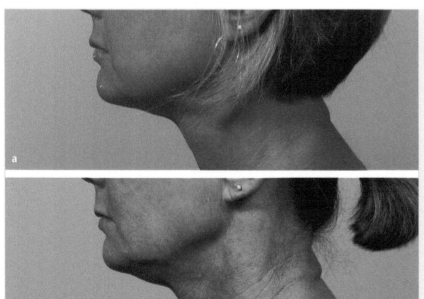

Fig. 14.1 (a) A 40-year-old woman. (b) Same patient at age 44. Both extrinsic and intrinsic aging has occurred.

While access ports under the earlobe and near the modiolus inside the mouth have been popular, there is a greater risk of burns and facial nerve weakness due to the awkward angle or long reach needed with these approaches. When treating the jowl, it is essential to treat behind and within the region, rather than trying to reach all the way to the chin. When near a known motor or sensory nerve site, it is wise to stay superficial, not too close, and for a very brief amount of time. If you see motor activity of the lower lip while treating, immediately cease treatment and go elsewhere.

14.5 Discussion

With aging, there is a diminishing collagenous stromal and vascular fraction in the soft tissue.[1] This is somewhat based on skin type, but the stronger factor is patient age. While it is well known that bone resorption, muscle atrophy, and atrophy of facial fat can result in a 200 cc facial volume loss over 30 years,[2] little attention has been paid to how the character of soft tissue changes. I would propose that the skin surface area probably does not increase with age. The combination of facial volume loss plus an increasing disconnect or "slide" between the soft tissue layers is the basic cause of facial contour changes with aging.[3] Volume loss is not the only factor influencing the apparent excess of the skin envelope. Strategically placed facial ligaments suspend facial skin, but the skin not anchored by these ligaments becomes flabby and loses tone over time as described above. ▶ Fig. 14.2 shows scanning electron micrographs of subcutaneous fat in patients of varying age. While there is not a linear division of soft tissue scaffold quality with age, it is generally a good predictor of how the fatty layer will behave. Several areas of the face known are known to be difficult to correct with traditional face lifting techniques.[4] The descent of the medial midface is marked by flattening of the upper cheek, and migration of that volume into the nasolabial fold region. By flattening the nasolabial fold with the RF device, the appearance of restoration of upper midface fullness can be achieved.

Another difficult region is the region of facial skin near the modiolus. A downturn of the mouth corners with age is almost universal, and is difficult to correct with surgery. The recreation of collagen support along with volume correction will significantly soften this marker of age.

A third target for focal RF correction is the region of soft tissue laxity just lateral to the marionette line (▶ Fig. 14.3). This slightly broader region is often characterized by superficial wrinkles and pendulosity when the patient is looking down. While wrinkle correction is better addressed by resurfacing, the

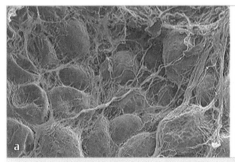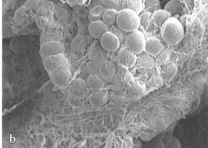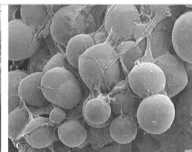

Fig. 14.2 Aging soft tissue. (**a**) 20s: prominent stromal and vascular component. (**b**) 40s: patchy areas of loss: both collagen-binding matrix and blood supply. (**c**) 60s: severely diminished stromal and vascular fraction.

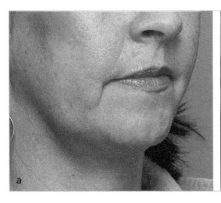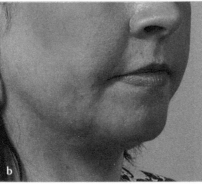

Fig. 14.3 (a) A 48-year-old prior to treatment. (b) 6 weeks post radiofrequency-assisted facelift and erbium laser resurfacing. Note the significant improvement of perioral "pouf" and jowl.

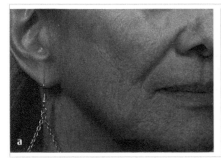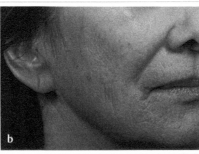

Fig. 14.4 Radiofrequency (RF) treatment alone. (a) 65-year-old prior to treatment. She declined any procedure that might look artificial or distorted. (b) Three weeks post-RF face lifting alone. Note significantly early jowl correction and perioral laxity. Skin tone and texture are also improved.

pendulosity can be well corrected with subcutaneous RF-assisted restoration of the collagen framework.

The fourth target in treating the central and lower midface is the jowl. This region is notoriously difficult to correct.[5,6] A complicating factor is the proximity of the marginal mandibular nerve. This branch of the facial nerve can be injured when exposed to thermal, physical, or chemical trauma.[7] Treatment of the jowl region with the RF device should be done very carefully, and in the region of the facial nerve, very superficially and briefly.

The root problem in the jowl is soft tissue (not skin) laxity behind the tight anchor of the mandibular ligament. Therefore, best correction would involve changing the character of the adipose layer, rather than pulling the overlying skin (facelift), or simply removing fat (liposuction). While micro-focused ultrasound[8] and injection lipolysis[9] have had moderate success in focal jowl treatment, consistent long term correction has been difficult to achieve.

The final target in treating the undercorrected aging face is the central submentum.[10] This may be the most difficult region to correct as no face or neck lifting method adequately corrects what appears to be skin laxity. In many cases, there is only a thin layer of fat associated with pendulous skin. The deformity is accentuated with a downward chin position. As long as some fat is present, the RF device, used with tumescent injection and only a few passes, can moderately tighten up this treatment-resistant area.

Patients should be warned that many of these regions show recurrent and/or residual aging easily. Softening, or possibly moderate improvement of these regions is all that should be expected with this RF assisted treatment. ▶Fig. 14.4 shows a rare patient who requested a minimal treatment as she desired no distortion or "look" of having had surgery. Early changes show improvement in the target area plus a surprising improvement in the appearance of the overlying skin.

14.6 Clinical Applications

The RF technique is ideal for many conditions other than simple soft tissue ptosis. While most patients request jowl correction along with improvement of submental laxity, many also note the descent of the fullest portion of the face from the central cheek to the nasolabial fold with time.

By flattening this protrusion, and creating linear "strands" of fibrosis from the nasolabial fold to the preauricular region, some facial suspension similar to that achieved with commercial suspension threads[11] or traditional surgical techniques[12] can be achieved.

Anther region satisfactorily treated include infraorbital malar bags and localized jowl laxity. Some women note perioral laxity with or without marionette lines. These are very difficult to treat. This region does respond well to RF lifting, but proximity to superficial facial nerve branches make this a region to be extremely careful with.

14.7 Combination Therapy

As with most surgical procedures, the outcomes are best when combined with other indicated procedures. Several common combinations include traditional facelift plus central RF assistance, short scar techniques with RF assistance, or combination with a brow lift to optimize the effect. A very effective combination is facial volume addition, skin resurfacing, and soft tissue tightening with this device. Obviously, you would add fat or fillers after the RF session, as melting of the filler or fat would be expected with the use of this device.

▶Fig. 14.5 shows preoperative markings in a patient who had midface laxity and prominent jowls. ▶Fig. 14.6 shows her preoperative appearance and postoperative result following a closed minimally invasive RF assisted facelift.

See ▶Table 14.1 for the pros and cons of Bipolar RF face lifting.

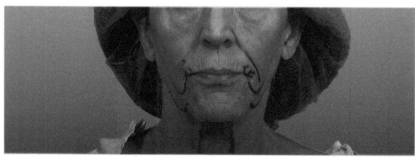

Fig. 14.5 Markings for radiofrequency treatment targets.

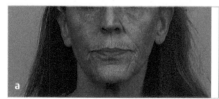
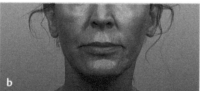

Fig. 14.6 Closed facelift result. (a) 63-year-old prior to treatment. (b) Patient 6 weeks following erbium laser resurfacing, fat grafting, and radiofrequency-assisted facelift.

Table 14.1 Pros and cons of bipolar radiofrequency face lifting

Pros	Cons
Scarless—no visible sign a procedure was performed	This approach limits the amount of correction that can be achieved
Addressing of focal problems is possible	Large problems may not be able to be improved fully
This procedure treats the basic cause of ptosis: soft tissue laxity	Significant facial reshaping is not possible
Downtime is minimal	But patient must wear support garment to optimize outcome
Small improvement visible right away	Optimal outcome takes 36 months to become evident

References

[1] Duncan DI, Kim TH, Temaat R. Quantification of adipose volume reduction with a prospective study analyzing the application of external radiofrequency energy and high voltage ultrashort pulse duration electrical fields. J Cosmet Laser Ther 2016;18(6):323–329

[2] Sadick NS, Dorizas AS, Krueger N, Nassar AH. The facial adipose system: its role in facial aging and approaches to volume restoration. Dermatol Surg 2015; 41(Suppl 1):S333–S339

[3] Duncan DI. Non-surgical treatments for the upper arm. 5CC conference, 2 Sept 2016, Barcelona

[4] Wan D, Small KH, Barton FE. Face lift. Plast Reconstr Surg 2015;136(5):676e–689e

[5] Jones BM, Lo SJ. How long does a face lift last? Objective and subjective measurements over a 5-year period. Plast Reconstr Surg 2012;130(6):1317–1327

[6] Narasimhan K, Stuzin JM, Rohrich RJ. Five-step neck lift: integrating anatomy with clinical practice to optimize results. Plast Reconstr Surg 2013;132(2):339–350

[7] Daane SP, Owsley JQ. Incidence of cervical branch injury with "marginal mandibular nerve pseudo-paralysis" in patients undergoing face lift. Plast Reconstr Surg 2003;111(7):2414–2418

[8] Wulkan AJ, Fabi SG, Green JB. Microfocused ultrasound for facial photorejuvenation: a review. Facial Plast Surg 2016;32(3):269–275

[9] Hasengschwandtner F. Injection lipolysis for effective reduction of localized fat in place of minor surgical lipoplasty. Aesthet Surg J 2006;26(2):125–130

[10] Rasko YM, Beale E, Rohrich RJ. Secondary rhytidectomy: comprehensive review and current concepts. Plast Reconstr Surg 2012;130(6):1370–8. Review

[11] Park TH, Seo SW, Whang KW. Facial rejuvenation with fine-barbed threads: the simple Miz lift. Aesthetic Plast Surg 2014;38(1):69–74

[12] Barrett DM, Gerecci D, Wang TD. Facelift controversies. Facial Plast Surg Clin North Am 2016;24(3):357–66. Review

15 Injection Lipolysis–Neck

Sachin M. Shridharani

Abstract

Injection adipocytolysis is a relatively new concept for treating discernable pockets of fat. Though injecting medications in the hope of destroying adipocytes has been ongoing for years, there has never been a Food and Drug Administration (FDA) approved drug for this aesthetic indication until the introduction of deoxycholic acid (ATX-101) into our aesthetic armamentarium. This treatment requires no incision or scar creation and its slight discomfort is ameliorated with pretreatment of local anesthetic injection. The irreversible destruction of the adipocytes leads to significant, bespoke, non-surgical contouring of the treated area.

Keywords: Injection adipocytolysis, ATX-101, submental fullness, jowls, face contouring, neck contouring, jawline contouring

---

Key Points

- FDA approved first in class drug to permanently destroy adipocytes and treat submental fullness.
- Non-selective cytolysis.
- Addition to aesthetic physician armamentarium to treat patients with palpable preplatysmal fat for neck contouring.

15.1 Introduction

A youthful appearing neck remains essential to the aesthetically pleasing face. The submental region/neck falls into the "lower third" of a full-face assessment and has a strong impact on the overall aesthetics of a male or female. Hallmarks of the ideal aesthetic neck are: distinct mandibular border, cervicomental angle of 105 to 120 degrees, visible anterior border of the sternocleidomastoid m., subhyoid depression, and thyroid cartilage bulge (▶Fig. 15.1).[1] All characteristics of the aesthetically pleasing neck can be softened or obliterated by accumulation of submental fat also known as the preplatysmal fat, resulting in an undefined and unpleasing neck appearance. Submental fat accumulation can be attributed to aging, obesity, poor lifestyle and diet, or genetic predisposition.[2,3] As stigmata of aging and/or obesity, an excess accumulation of subcutaneous fat in the neck may have negative psychological impact.

Several multimodal approaches to neck rejuvenation have been employed to address unwanted submental fat. Invasive techniques, including platysmaplasty, liposuction, direct lipectomy, or any combination of these procedures can be effective in addressing submental fat.[1,4] These procedures may not be suitable or desired by all patients, however. Invasive procedures, while generally well-tolerated, have: increased recovery times, higher risk profile, need for additional staff expertise, need for anesthesia, and need for additional office infrastructure—operating room or similar suite. Several of the technical considerations resultantly lead to increased procedural costs. Non-surgical energy devices have been developed to address excess submental fat are limited by insufficient evidence supporting their efficacy.

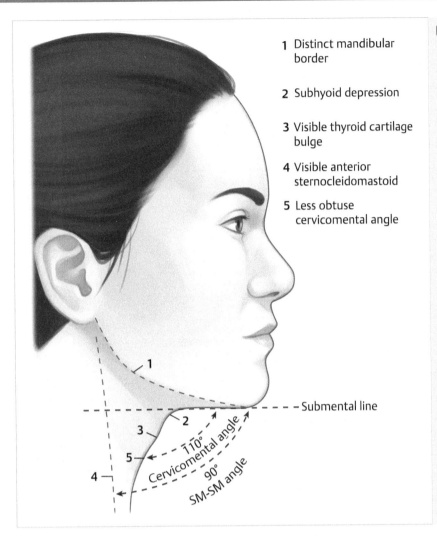

Fig. 15.1 Youthful neck.

1 Distinct mandibular border

2 Subhyoid depression

3 Visible thyroid cartilage bulge

4 Visible anterior sternocleidomastoid

5 Less obtuse cervicomental angle

The need for an effective, noninvasive alternative to surgical management of excess submental fat was the impetus to the development of the injectable form of the lipolytic agent deoxycholic acid (DCA). The drug was studied under the name: ATX-101. To date the only FDA approved agent of the market is Kybella (Allergan Pharmaceuticals, Irvine, California) (▶Fig. 15.1).

15.2 Deoxycholic Acid (DCA)

Over the last several decades, chemical techniques for fat reduction have been developed as nonsurgical alternatives. The first agent utilized was phosphatidylcholine (PC), introduced in 1985 for the treatment of xanthelasmas. Later, PC was used for correction of lower eyelid bulging due to prominent fat pads[5,6] and for localized subcutaneous fat deposits.[7,8] With further experience, it was observed that DCA, the solvent for PC, was responsible for the lytic action of PC/DCA combination formulations on cells in cell culture and fresh porcine skin, leading to the hypothesis that detergents play a role in the elimination of undesired adipose tissue. Studies demonstrated that DCA-alone induced adipose cell lysis just as effectively as DCA with PC.[9]

Deoxycholic acid is a naturally occurring, bile-derived compound found in most animals[10] and functions as a nonselective detergent-like lipolytic agent.[11] Detergents have both hydrophobic and hydrophilic regions and are classified as ionic, nonionic, or zwitterionic.[12] Sodium deoxycholate belongs to the ionic group of detergents, containing polar and nonpolar chemical properties that function to emulsify insoluble substances by reducing surface tension of cell membranes.[12,13] In doing so, DCA causes adipocyte rupture by disrupting the integrity of adipocyte cell membranes, which results in smaller micelles of fat that ultimately undergo phagocytosis. The DCA is in turn metabolized through the liver while the remaining adipocyte remnants are excreted through the gastrointestinal tract.

When injected into the subcutaneous layer, DCA causes adipocyte lysis ultimately resulting in decreased adipocyte density with fibrotic tissue replacing the adipose tissue.[12] The resulting physical and histological changes do not lead to atrophy or hardening of the surface layer of the skin, but rather has been hypothesized to instigate a moderate skin tightening/retracting effect. These combined effects have led to increasing public interest in DCA as an ideal substance for minimally invasive treatment of unwanted fat.

15.3 Patient Evaluation

Assessment of the neck for lipolytic injectable treatment requires a thorough understanding of preplatysmal fat and its compartmentalization. As in other fat compartments of the face, the submental fat pad is located in a distinct compartment. Housed within the preplatysmal fat, the submental fat pad is consolidated to the submental crease, caudal continuation of labiomandibular fold, and palpable hyoid bone. The fullness can contribute to an obtuse cervicomental angle (▶Fig. 15.2).[14] There exists a continuation of submental fat pad outside the anatomic landmarks, however, the fat is less full (generally) but is uniformly distributed in the subcutaneous space. In cadaveric studies, the dispersion of injections of dyed gelatin was used to elucidate the boundaries of submental fat compartments.[15] Injection of lipolytics can be expected to disperse similarly and understanding this compartmental anatomy is essential in procedural planning to address specific patient needs. On initial patient evaluation, the submental landmarks should be identified and the contained soft tissue evaluated with special attention toward volume, contour, skin quality and thickness, and any preexisting asymmetries (▶Fig. 15.2).

Patient evaluation and physical exam are quite straightforward and mirror evaluation of patients who are requesting liposuction in this anatomic area. The physical exam maneuvers require the physician to pinch, palpate, pull, and have patient grimace. Pinching and palpating allows one to assess the amount of palpable subcutaneous fat in this region. An obtuse cervicomental

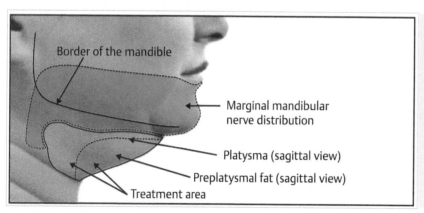

Border of the mandible

Marginal mandibular nerve distribution

Platysma (sagittal view)

Preplatysmal fat (sagittal view)

Treatment area

Fig. 15.2 Aging neck with submental fullness.

angle could also be secondary to platysma laxity and aging skin with minimal submental fullness (SMF). Care should be taken to rule out thyroid goiter, neck masses, adenopathy, and prominent submandibular glands. Once the practitioner establishes that there is presence of subcutaneous fat amenable to treatment, pulling on the skin and looking for laxity and dermal recoil helps the physician establish whether or not the patient is a good candidate. Ideally, the patient has appropriate skin recoil, which establishes that he/she will benefit from the treatment and see significant improvement from the subsequent fibrosis, which results after the liquefactive necrosis is cleared during the inflammatory reaction. Finally, asking the patient to grimace effectively is asking the patient to fire his/her platysma muscle which forces the post-platysma fat deep allowing the practitioner to assess the subcutaneous fat of the neck. One can liken this maneuver to asking patients to fire his/her rectus abdominis muscles, which pushes intra-abdominal fat deep and allows one to only pinch and palpate the subcutaneous fat of the abdomen.

15.4 Preoperative Planning and Preparation

Patients should undergo physical and local examination (assessment for edema, bruising, numbness, paresis, and tenderness), assessment of vital signs, and evaluation for bleeding disorders before and after initiation of each treatment session. The only absolute contraindication to the procedure is active infection at the treatment site. The patient should be counseled that he/she will experience a period of edema secondary to the inflammatory response. The swelling can be pronounced, but generally fully resolves by day 5–10 depending on age, skin laxity, amount of subcutaneous fat, and aggressive nature of treatment (amount of medication used).

Pre-procedure photography should be undertaken to document response. Respecting the Frankfort horizontal plane is critical to standardize angles of the photos. The patient should be counseled that he or she should anticipate the need for 2–4 treatments at 6 weeks intervals to see full effect. Furthermore, there is continued improvement without treatment at weeks 6–12 during wound healing.

15.5 Surgical Technique (▶ Fig. 15.3a–k)

Treatment with deoxycholic acid is generally performed as a semi-sterile procedure. The patient's submental region can be prepped with standard alcohol wipes prior to marking.

15.5.1 Positioning and Markings

The patient is marked in the sitting upright position and care should be exercised to avoid the marginal mandibular zone of innervation in the planned and marked treatment area. Once initial markings are in place, it may be prudent to review the location and nature of the injections with the patient to ensure optimized contouring and to best address the specific patient's needs. The patient is then assisted into the reclined position for application of a grid, which comes with each medication kit. Using the grid is imperative as the markings are equally spaced 1 cm apart. The diffusion zone of Kybella in the subcutaneous space is 1 cm.[2] Injecting at the appropriate grid location ensures

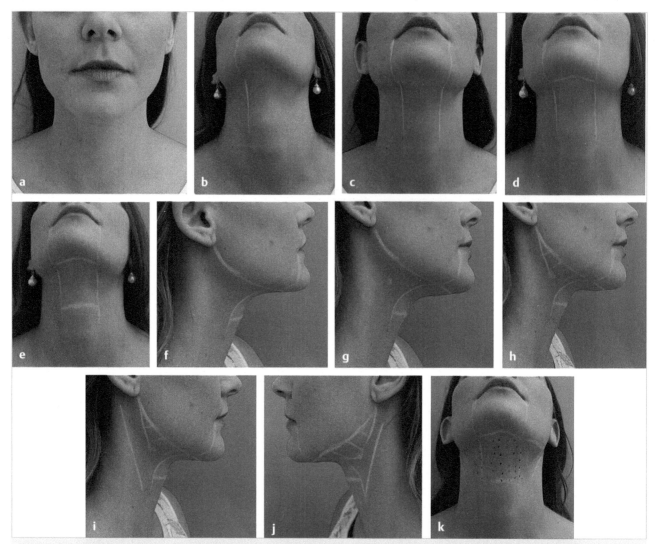

Fig. 15.3 Kybella markings. (**a**) Clean the surface of the skin with antiseptic of choice. The senior author favors utilizing standard isopropyl alcohol. (**b**) Utilizing a marking pencil, the right labiomandibular fold is identified at the oral commissure and continued in a caudal fashion to lateral of the thyroid cartilage. (**c**) The left labiomandibular fold is identified at the oral commissure and continued in a caudal fashion to lateral of the thyroid cartilage. (**d**) The submental crease is identified and marked from one labiomandibular line to the contralateral line. (**e**) The thyroid cartilage is noted and a horizontal line is delineated from the caudal extensions of the labiomandibular lines. (**f**) A line is marked from the right ear lobule to the submental crease along the inferior aspect of the mandibular border. (**g**) A point is located 2.5 cm below the line drawn in Step 6 halfway between the ear lobule and the center of the chin. (**h**) A curvilinear line is drawn from the ear lobule through the point drawn in Step 7 and connected to the submental line. This is the approximate location of the marginal mandibular nerve and should not be injected (*hash marks*). (**i**) The patient is asked to turn his/ her head to the contralateral side to cause the sternocleidomastoid muscle to bulge. A line is drawn along the anterior border of the muscle. No treatments should occur posterior to this line. (**j**) Steps 6–9 are performed on the contralateral side. (**k**) The included spacing grid is applied with a wet sponge or gauze (sterile water). Care is taken to place the top of the grid (short side) against the submental crease. Remove grid points that do not fall in the markings with alcohol wipes.

there is equal distribution and diffusion of the medication such that the adipo-cytes are bathed appropriately leading to a uniform treatment. Once reclined, the grid is applied with gauze soaked with sterile water. Once applied, any grid points that do not fall into the marked zone of treatment are removed with alcohol wipes (▶Fig. 15.4).

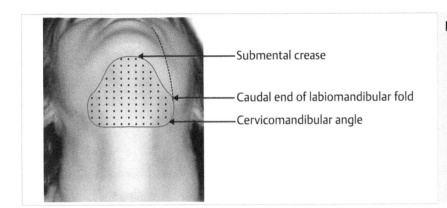

Fig. 15.4 Grid application.

Submental crease

Caudal end of labiomandibular fold

Cervicomandibular angle

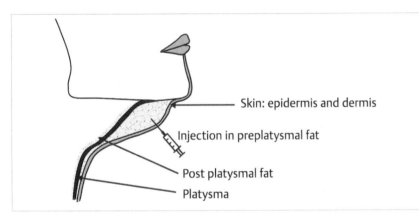

Fig. 15.5 Injection location (sagittal view).

Skin: epidermis and dermis

Injection in preplatysmal fat

Post platysmal fat

Platysma

15.5.2 Anesthesia

The procedure does not require any anesthesia, however, the use of local anesthetics can be very helpful. At the bare minimum, it is heavily advised to employ the use of ice prior to injection and directly after the procedure. The benefits would include local numbing and vasoconstriction, which leads to decreased bruising and overall comfort during these injections. Use of topical anesthetics can be beneficial, however, are not necessary since the submental skin is not particularly sensitive to small injections. Use of injectable local anesthetics can be very helpful and are often employed to decrease the discomfort associated with the immediate adipocyte destruction from the deoxycholic acid induced cell membrane rupture. The authors favor using 1% or 2% lidocaine with epinephrine 1:100,000 infiltrated subcutaneously into the desired zone of treatment. Generally, 4–8 cc of local anesthetic are more than sufficient to obtain appropriate anesthesia.

15.5.3 Technique

A total of 0.2 cc/cm is injected subcutaneously at each grid point. The injection is optimized by using a 0.5 inch 30 g v 32 g hypodermic needle. Needle penetration 1/2 to 2/3 the length of the needle, ensures that one is in the subcutaneous space and not deep dermal (▶ Fig. 15.5). Use of cannulas is discouraged, as one cannot accurately place the medication at each injection point. The grid points are then removed with alcohol wipes and an ice pack is promptly placed over the injected area.

15.6 Results and Outcomes

Deoxycholic acid (ATX-101) was FDA approved in 2015 in the United States (Kybella) and Canada (Belkyra) for treatment of submental fullness to improve the appearance of moderate to severe convexity. To date, there have been several successful multi-institutional, randomized-controlled phase 3 trials evaluating the efficacy and safety profile of DCA.[6,7,8,9] In the REFINE-1 phase 3 clinical trial, the investigators assessed both clinical response, MRI volumetric response, as well as psychological impact of ATX-101 treatment in 256 patients.[6] They report 75% of patients undergoing 4 treatments had a 1-grade improvement in submental fat (e.g., from severe to moderate, or from moderate to mild SMF). Further, compared to placebo, ATX-101 treated patients had an 8-fold greater proportion who had reduction in SMF fat (defined as >10% reduction in SMF from baseline) on MRI interrogation. These volumetric changes have previously been described as clinically meaningful to patients in phase 2 studies, and were associated with a positive visual- and emotional self-perceptions.[6]

15.6.1 Case 1

A 24-year-old female presented to the office with a desire to get rid of her "double chin"(▶Fig. 15.4). She states that irrespective of how well she eats or how much she exercises, she is unable to achieve a better-defined jawline and "cleaner" neckline. She mentions that her mother has the "same neck" and is not obese. The patient has no history of any surgical procedures and is afraid of undergoing elective surgery. She requests a treatment that will improve the appearance of this area with significant control by the physician and not just get rid of "bulk." She has no history of cervical adenopathy or thyroid goiter.

On exam, the patient has palpable subcutaneous fat in the submental region. No evidence of skin laxity or platysma muscle diastasis. When grimacing (activating platysma muscle), there is no visible sign or palpable evidence of post-platysma fat being drawn away. She does not have prominent submandibular glands. There is no evidence of scarring in the area.

She is pictured one day pre-injection (▶Fig. 15.6a, c). She underwent two treatments with Kybella (2 mg/cm) spaced 2 months apart. A robust result is shown 2 months after her second treatment (▶Fig. 15.6b, d). She was very satisfied with her result (▶Fig. 15.6a–d).

15.6.2 Case 2

A 55-year-old male presented to the office with a desire to get rid of his "double chin (▶Fig. 15.5)." He states that he notes excess skin and fullness despite youthful body appearance. He does not want any surgical intervention for his face. He has no history of cervical adenopathy, thyroid goiter or prominent submandibular glands.

On exam, the patient has palpable subcutaneous fat in the submental region. There is moderate skin laxity, but no platysma muscle diastasis. When grimacing there is no visible sign or palpable evidence of post-platysma fat being drawn away. There is no evidence of scarring in the area.

Patient is pictured one day pre-injection (left side) and after undergoing two treatments with Kybella (2 mg/cm) spaced 6 weeks apart (right side). Results

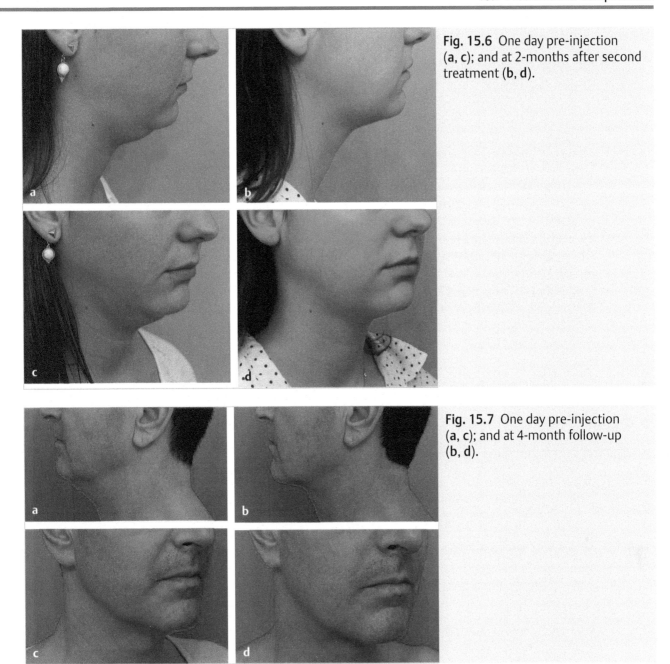

Fig. 15.6 One day pre-injection (**a, c**); and at 2-months after second treatment (**b, d**).

Fig. 15.7 One day pre-injection (**a, c**); and at 4-month follow-up (**b, d**).

are shown 4 months after his second treatment. He was very pleased with this result (▶ Fig. 15.7).

15.7 Problems and Complications

Deoxycholic acid has been demonstrated in clinical trials in the United States to be both safe and effective to decrease SMF secondary to presence of excess subcutaneous fat.[16] While generally well tolerated and a safe alternative to surgical interventions, deoxycholic acid lipolysis is not without its own complications and limitations. Caution should be exercised during each treatment session due to the non-selective cytolytic nature of deoxycholic acid. DCA action is attenuated by protein-binding in non-lipid rich environments, limiting unintended vertical penetration beyond muscular borders in the treatment of SMF. Understanding the anticipated horizontal distribution of DCA after injection and ensuring proper needle placement guided by an understanding of fat compartmentalization becomes essential. Because the lytic effects of deoxycholic acid are dose related, studies systematically evaluating treatment response based on concentration and volume of deoxycholic acid at injection site are still required to avoid adverse response. Current and appropriate treatment regimen is staying "on label" with the product. Kybella's formulation is 1% DCA. Injection of less than 2 mg/cm leads to a sub-therapeutic response. Interestingly, injecting greater than 2 mg/cm leads to similar sub-therapeutic response and not even a plateau effect based on pharmacologic studies. This is important so in an attempt to decrease swelling physicians should not treat with less medication and greater treatments, since each treatment will effectively be sub-therapeutic. Furthermore, utilizing more medication in a single setting in hopes of limiting treatment number will also lead to patient dissatisfaction and sub-therapeutic response and higher risk profile.

In the FDA studies, local edema/swelling (87%), bruising (72%), pain (70%), and numbness (66%) were the most common side effects. Less commonly, erythema (27%), induration (23%), or temporary marginal mandibular nerve dysfunction (4%) was encountered.[13,17,18] Marginal mandibular nerve dysfunction is a complication of particular interest, as it can cause transient asymmetry. In the REFINE-1 clinical trial, the observed rate of marginal mandibular dysfunction was 4%, or 1.0% per treatment session.[17] This has been reflected in other clinical trials.[19,20,21,22] In all studies, the effect on marginal mandibular nerve function was transient. In this author's own subsequent prospective, single-institution study of 100 consecutive patients, it was observed that mean duration of swelling was 7.7 days, numbness 28.5 days, and pain 3.5 days.

Current literature suggests that the initial use of low-dose deoxycholic acid followed by close and routine patient follow-up is important for managing reactions and adverse events and further patient expectations. Patient follow-up is likely to vary; patients might prefer to undergo this procedure during winter months when clothing can hide transient swelling and redness. Increasing the number of injections per session for the same total dose and avoiding injection into the skin may reduce local scarring, ulceration, and fibrosis.

Further, as with any injectable, deoxycholic acid cannot fully address deformity more amenable to invasive surgical options. These include patients with significant ptosis secondary to soft tissue support attenuation in the aging face or in the massive weight-loss patient. Patient selection remains key. The ideal patients for injection lipolysis are those with excess adiposity of the submental area with preserved skin elasticity and support integrity. It has been postulated that DCA does have a modest effect on skin contraction, as studies demonstrating volume decreases after treatment did not also demonstrate any increase in laxity as one might otherwise expect.[19,20] While DCA may effect improvement even in the setting of some ptosis, pre-existing excess skin cannot be corrected by lipolysis alone. In these circumstances, lipolysis should be used in conjunction with other noninvasive skin tightening modalities,[23] or as an adjunct to traditional surgical neck rejuvenation techniques.[24] Appropriate utilization of injection lipolysis in the appropriate patient remains key.

References

[1] Co AC, Abad-Casintahan MF, Espinoza-Thaebtharm A. Submental fat reduction by meso-therapy using phosphatidylcholine alone vs. phosphatidylcholine and organic silicium: a pilot study. J Cosmet Dermatol 2007;6(4):250–257

[2] Duncan DI, Chubaty R. Clinical safety data and standards of practice for injection lipolysis: a retrospective study. Aesthet Surg J 2006;26(5):575–585

[3] Patel BC. Aesthetic surgery of the aging neck: options and techniques. Orbit 2006;25(4):327–356

[4] Koehler J. Complications of neck liposuction and submentoplasty. Oral Maxillofac Surg Clin North Am 2009;21(1):43–52, vi.

[5] Rittes PG. The use of phosphatidylcholine for correction of lower lid bulging due to prominent fat pads. Dermatol Surg 2001;27(4):391–392

[6] Ablon G, Rotunda AM. Treatment of lower eyelid fat pads using phosphatidylcholine: clinical trial and review. Dermatol Surg 2004;30(3):422–427, discussion 428

[7] Rittes PG. The use of phosphatidylcholine for correction of localized fat deposits. Aesthetic Plast Surg 2003;27(4):315–318

[8] Young VL. Lipostabil: the effect of phosphatidylcholine on subcutaneous fat. Aesthet Surg J 2003;23(5):413–417

[9] Rotunda AM, Weiss SR, Rivkin LS. Randomized double-blind clinical trial of subcutaneously injected deoxycholate versus a phosphatidylcholine-deoxycholate combination for the reduction of submental fat. Dermatol Surg 2009;35(5):792–803

[10] Tanner B, Barabas T, Crook D, Link C. A future for injection lipolysis? Aesthet Surg J 2013;33(3):456–457

[11] Salti G, Rauso R. Comments on Injection lipolysis with phosphatidylcholine and deoxycholate. Aesthet Surg J 2014;34(4):639–640

[12] Yagima Odo ME, Cucé LC, Odo LM, Natrielli A. Action of sodium deoxycholate on subcutaneous human tissue: local and systemic effects. Dermatol Surg 2007;33(2):178–188, discussion 188–189

[13] Rotunda AM, Suzuki H, Moy RL, Kolodney MS. Detergent effects of sodium deoxycholate are a major feature of an injectable phosphatidylcholine formulation used for localized fat dissolution. Dermatol Surg 2004;30(7):1001–1008

[14] ASPS. Top 5 Procedures in 2015, <http://www.plasticsurgery.org/news/plastic-surgery-statistics.html> (2015)

[15] Pilsl U, Anderhuber F. The chin and adjacent fat compartments. Dermatol Surg 2010;36(2):214–218

[16] Dayan SH, Arkins JP, Chaudhry R. Minimally invasive neck lifts: have they replaced neck lift surgery? Facial Plast Surg Clin North Am 2013;21(2):265–270

[17] Jones DH, Carruthers J, Joseph JH, et al. REFINE-1, a Multicenter, Randomized, Double-Blind, Placebo-Controlled, Phase 3 Trial With ATX-101, an Injectable Drug for Submental Fat Reduction. Dermatol Surg 2016;42(1):38–49

[18] Cohen JL, Chen DL, Green JB, Joseph JH. Additional thoughts on the new treatment Kybella. Semin Cutan Med Surg 2015;34(3):138–139

[19] Rzany B, Griffiths T, Walker P, Lippert S, McDiarmid J, Havlickova B. Reduction of unwanted submental fat with ATX-101 (deoxycholic acid), an adipocytolytic injectable treatment: results from a phase III, randomized, placebo-controlled study. Br J Dermatol 2014;170(2):445–453

[20] Ascher B, Hoffmann K, Walker P, Lippert S, Wollina U, Havlickova B. Efficacy, patient-reported outcomes and safety profile of ATX-101 (deoxycholic acid), an injectable drug for the reduction of unwanted submental fat: results from a phase III, randomized, placebo-controlled study. J Eur Acad Dermatol Venereol 2014;28(12):1707–1715

[21] Walker P, Lee D. A phase 1 pharmacokinetic study of ATX-101: serum lipids and adipokines following synthetic deoxycholic acid injections. J Cosmet Dermatol 2015;14(1):33–39

[22] Kybella. https://www.accessdata.fda.gov/drugsatfda_docs/label/2018/206333s001lbl.pdf

[23] Vanaman M, Fabi SG, Cox SE. Neck Rejuvenation Using a Combination Approach: Our Experience and a Review of the Literature. Dermatol Surg 2016;42(Suppl 2):S94–S100

[24] Rohrich RJ, Ghavami A, Constantine FC, Unger J, Mojallal A. Lift-and-fill face lift: integrating the fat compartments. Plast Reconstr Surg 2014;133(6):756e–767e

16 Neck: Radiofrequency Liposuction

Evangelos Keramidas

Abstract

Radiofrequency-assisted liposuction (RFAL) is a relatively new technology which is based on the delivery of direct radiofrequency energy into the subcutaneous fat achieving simultaneously coagulation, fat dissociation, and collagen contracture. RFAL can be performed under local anesthesia in a varieties of body areas. In this chapter, we describe the use of RFAL for treatment of the neck area which is one of the most difficult areas to treat. RFAL the last year acquired FDA approval.

Keywords: Radiofrequency-assisted liposuction, neck contouring, neck tightening, face contouring, new technology

> **Key Points**
>
> - RFAL is a relatively new technique that applies radiofrequency energy to soft tissues in a bipolar manner.
> - RFAL can offer significant skin contraction to the neck and body area.
> - RFAL could be used effectively to achieve long-lasting non-excisional neck skin tightening and face contouring.
> - The most common side effects is temporary in duration and firmness of the soft tissue of the neck and superficial burns.

16.1 Introduction

The cervical region and face contour are some of the most challenging anatomic areas and difficult to aesthetically correct.

Face and neck lift is the gold standard treatment for correction of skin laxity of the neck. However, these techniques leave the patient with scars and long recovery time.

The non-excisional improvement of the face and neck contour remains a challenging problem and the noninvasive or minimally invasive techniques gain much popularity day by day.

RFAL technology has been widely applied over the last years with promising results in several areas of the body.[1,2,3,4,5,6] Peer-reviewed articles show skin contracture of up to 34% over 12 months period with very satisfactory and long-lasting aesthetic results.[2]

16.2 Patient Selection

Best candidates for the treatment are patients of type I and type II neck irregularities, according to the Baker classification are as follows:[7]
- Type I: Slight cervical skin laxity with submental fat and early jowls.
- Type II: Moderate cervical skin laxity, moderate jowls, and submental fat.
- Type III: Moderate cervical skin laxity, but with significant jowling and active platysmal banding.
- Type IV: Loose redundant cervical skin and folds below the cricoid, significant jowls, and active platysmal bands.

16.3 Preoperative Planning and Preparation

The procedure can be performed under local anesthesia (LA), or LA and sedation whereas for patients that are combined with other procedures (blepharoplasty, facelift etc.), general anesthesia is recommended. Prophylactic intravenous antibiotic is administered half an hour before the operation. Prophylactic antithrombotic stockings and sequentially compression stockings are applied to all patients. Temperature of the operating room is maintained at 22°C.

Continuous pulse oximetry and intermittent blood pressure monitoring is recorded in all patients during surgery and recovery.

Patient is marked in a standing position. For patients above 40 years old we check EGG, full blood count, blood clotting test, liver function test, kidney test, and chest X-ray.

Patients are requested to give up any herbal or supplement which could increase the chances for hematoma two weeks before and two weeks after the treatment.

Patients who are excluded are as follows: Under 16 years of age and above 70 years old, history of medication taking that may increase bleeding, pregnancy, lactation, high expectations, history of liver or kidney failure, patients with pacemaker, previous scarring in the neck, history of blood clotting problems, heart disease, history of diabetes, loss of weight <40 kg.

16.4 Surgical Technique

16.4.1 Marking the Neck

The neck is divided into three zones (▶ Fig. 16.1) one medially (I) and two laterally (II, III). The central zone I is the area between the right and left tracheal gutter. The lateral zones II and III extent from the medial border of the sternocleidomastoid muscle to the jawline and the lateral tracheal gutter. We apply the RFAL handpiece separately to each area.

16.5 Incisions

Three stab incisions are used. These incisions are performed with 11 blades. One submental incision and two sub-lobular.

16.6 Infiltration

A 14-G infiltration cannula is used to deliver the infiltration solution that consists of 1.5 mg adrenaline 1:1000, 50 mgr lidocaine 2% and 10 cc bicarbonate. The solution is delivered to the subcutaneous tissue until sufficient turgor is achieved.

After 15–20 minutes of waiting for the vasoconstriction effect of the adrenaline, we begin the operation.

16.7 Devices

The RFAL is performed with the bodyTite device (Invasix, Yoki-nem, Israel). The bodyTite system uses an RF generator and a handpiece bipolar RF which delivers the RF frequency and heat internally to the adipose tissue. The RF

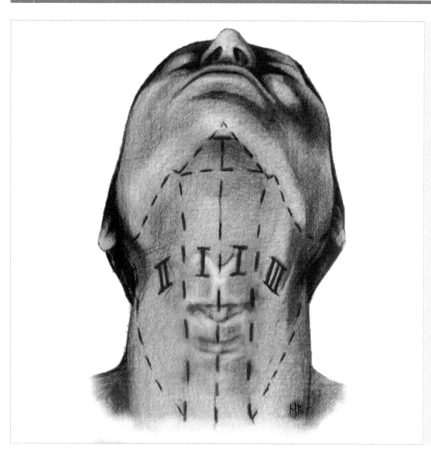

Fig. 16.1 Marking the neck.

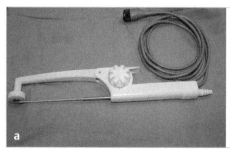
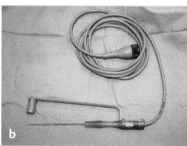

Fig. 16.2 (a) Necktite handpiece. (b) Facetite hadpiece.

generator provides continuous skin temperature measurements with a negative feedback loop control of power.

In the neck we use two devices: the necktite cannula (▶Fig. 16.2a) and the facetite handpiece (▶Fig. 16.2b).

The necktite hand piece is 12 cm of length and with diameter of 24 mm. There is also a hole for fat aspiration in this cannula. The facetite handpiece is of 10 cm length, 17 mm diameter and is a solid non-aspiration bipolar RF device for sub-dermal coagulative heating and transdermal non-ablative RF skin tightening. There is no hole in this device.

The necktite cannula, delivers the bipolar radiofrequency energy, which is internally coagulative and externally non-ablative bulk heating. Coagulation, deep FSN contraction, and soft-tissue tightening and the external electrode glides along the skin surface in coordination with the internal electrode, receiving RF from the internal electrode and delivering non-ablative skin heating and tightening. The device has an external thermistor, high and low impedance and no contact sensors and will turn off the RF when the therapeutic target temperature has been reached, or if there are potentially dangerous high or low tissue impedance readings, or loss of epidermal contact.[8,9,10]

16.8 Gel

Zones I, II, and III are covered with sterile ultrasound gel to facilitate the movement of the devices and improve RF delivery.

16.9 Technique

The RF Power setting is 15 watts and the epidermal cut off temperature is set to 38°C. When the temperature of 38°C is reached, the RF energy is automatically cut off. The moment the soft tissue temperature is 0.1°C. below 38°C, the RF energy is automatically turned on again. This automatic feedback loop of target temperature controlled Radiofrequency allows the surgeon to maintain uniform tissue temperature for prolonged periods of time. We continue the treatment on each area for 1 minute continuously, once the thermal endpoint has been reached. For the facetite applicators, the power of RF is 10 watts and cut off temperature is again set at 38°C.

The thermal stimulation of the upper dermis and shortening effect to the fibrous septal network[8,9,10] contribute to collagen contraction and soft tissue tightening in a degree that even severe skin laxity can be treated safely in the sub-mental area adjacent regions. In addition, the embedded thermal sensor within the external electrode achieves a more targeted and uniform temperature distribution without any red spots and a reduced risk of thermal injuries or untreated areas such as those found in laser-assisted liposuction.[11,12]

16.10 Depth of the Treatment

The depth of treatment is controlled by choosing the distance between the two electrodes prior to the operation adjusting the desired level. We treat the area of the neck at the level of 5 or 6. We believe that delivering smaller energy (w) and to the deeper tissues is reducing the possibilities for tissue hardening, yet still optimizes the contraction of the very important fibroseptal network (FSN).[1]

16.11 Surgical Tips

The internal RF-active electrode inserted inside infiltrated adipose tissue and deliver RF energy and heat internally to the adipose tissue. The external large-area electrode is applied just opposite to the internal electrode on the epidermal side.

The device is moved continuously in a back and forth motion to avoid any "hot spots."

During treatment the bodyTite device emits an audible double beep when the temperature is within 2°C of the cut off temperature and a triple beep when the cut-off temperature has been reached.

The central part of the neck (zone I) is held continuously on a hyperextended position when we perform RFAL to this area. Because of the concavity of zone I this is the most difficult area to be treated. The neck needs

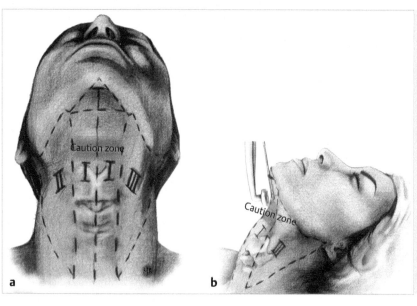

Fig. 16.3 (a, b) Schematic representation of the difficult zone for treatment. The neck needs to be hyperextended.

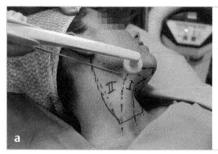
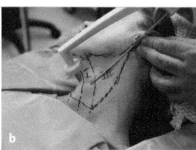

Fig. 16.4 (a) Treatment zone II. **(b)** Treatment zone III.

to be over-extended as much as possible in order to avoid a full thickness burn (►Fig. 16.3a, b).

For the treatment of zone II the patient is hyper-extended left and for the treatment of zone III the neck is hyper-extended to the right. (►Fig. 16.4a, b).

In very thin necks we treat the central part of the neck with the facetite handpiece using 10 KJ RF energy in order to avoid skin damage (burns).

For the final touches after the RF treatment we suction the emulsified fat immediately after the end of RF treatment. We use a 3 mm diameter spatula type with one hole cannula to obtain a thinner and uniformly thick fat layer. With pinch test we confirm the uniformity and the evenness of the skin.

After treatment, each incision is closed with 5–0 nylon for 5 days.

16.12 Statistics

The average necktite operative time is 45' (1 hour–25 minutes). The average total aspirated fat volume is 30 mL (200–10 cc). The average time for the lower face facetite (except for head and eyes) is 15'.

The RFAL delivers RF converted into heat, estimated in Kilojoules. The mean amount of energy delivered is 4,5 KJ/procedure (8.5–2 KJ).

16.13 Postoperative Care

A face and neck compression garment is recommended to be worn for 2 days. Patient can go to work the next day. There is no restriction to their daily routine.

16.14 Results

The criteria for a youthful neck as described by Ellanbogen et al are: a cervicomental angle of 105 to 120°, visible thyroid cartilage, well-defined interior mandibular border, a visible anterior sternocleidomastoid border, a visible subhyoid depression. Also, the existence or absence of labiomandibular fold prominence is very important for the youthful appearance of the neck[13,14] (▶Fig. 16.5).

Based on the above mentioned criteria and according to our continuing experience and our published results,[1] three independent plastic surgeons, familiar with neck rejuvenation procedures, scored the 6 month cervicomental and/or lower facial outcomes as moderate–excellent in 90% of the cases, whereas poor contour results in 10% of the cases. Moreover, 85% of the patients were satisfied or extremely satisfied 6 months following the RFAL non-excisional neck contour tightening, while 15% were dissatisfied with the degree of soft tissue contraction.

The majority of patients returned to work in 1–2 days.

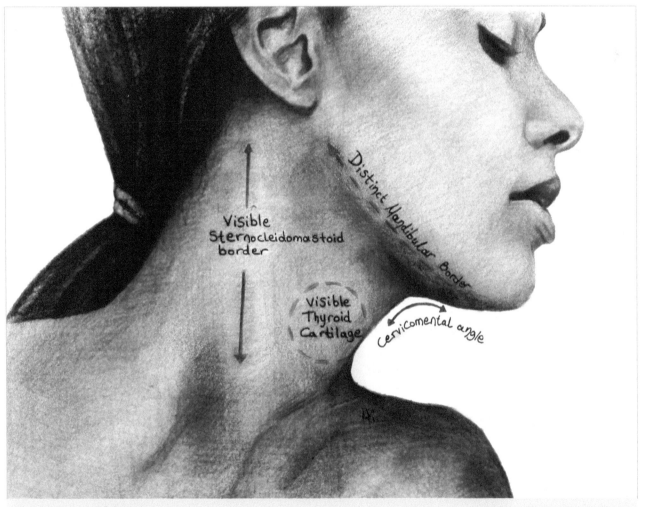

Fig. 16.5 Youthful neck.

16.15 Complications

There are no major complications with this technique. There is a small change of thermal injury which can be treated with local wound care.

Hardness of the subcutaneous tissue of the neck, can be observed which dissolve in 2–3 months. Transient paralysis (paresis) of the marginal mandibular branch of the facial nerve, is rare.

16.16 Case Studies

16.16.1 Case 1 (▶ Figs. 16.6a, c and 16.7a, c)

A 32-year-old woman with slight skin laxity and submental adipose tissue. Baker type I:
- Anesthesia: Local and sedation.
- Device Necktite: Power 15 W; cut off temperature 38°C; total energy delivered 5 KJ.
- Surgical time: 50 minutes.
- Fat aspiration: 105 mL.

Results

- Remarkable improvement of the neck.
- Patient extremely happy.

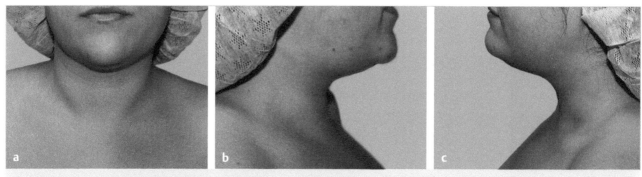

Fig. 16.6 Case 1. Preoperative picture (a) frontal view (b) right lateral view (c) left lateral view.

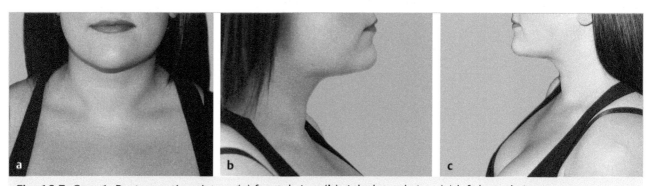

Fig. 16.7 Case 1. Postoperative picture (a) frontal view (b) right lateral view (c) left lateral view.

16.16.2 Case 2

A 44 year-old lady with moderate lax skin, jowls, obtuse cervicomental angle (Baker II) (►Fig. 16.8a, b and ►Fig. 16.9 a, b)
• Treatment of neck and lower face.
• Anesthesia: Local and sedation.
• Device Necktite: Power 15 W; cut off temperature 38°C; total energy delivered 6 KJ.
• Device Facetite: Power 15 W; cut off temperature 38°C; total energy delivered 1, 5 KJ.
• Total energy: 7, 5 KJ.
• Surgical time: 1 hour.

Results

Very good improvement of the neck and jowls.

16.16.3 Case 3

55-year-old male patient with moderate to severe severe laxity of the neck (Baker type II to III) (►Fig. 16.10a–c and ►Fig. 16.11a–c). Not a very good candidate for this technique however, the patient was informed of the limits of the technique and agreed to go ahead.
• Treatment of lower face also.
• Anesthesia: Local + sedation.
• Device Necktite: Power 15 W; cut off temperature 38°C; and total energy delivered 8 KJ.

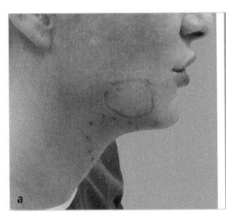
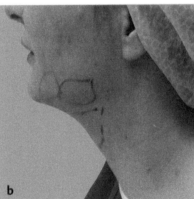

Fig. 16.8 Case 2. Preoperative picture (**a**) right lateral view (**b**) left lateral view.

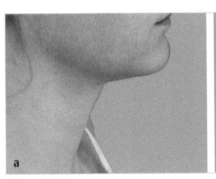
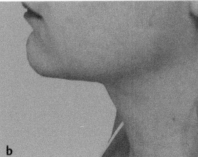

Fig. 16.9 Case 2. Postoperative picture (**a**) right lateral view (**b**) left lateral view.

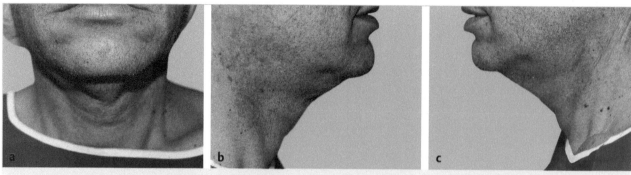

Fig. 16.10 Case 3. Preoperative picture (**a**) frontal view (**b**) right lateral view (**c**) left lateral view.

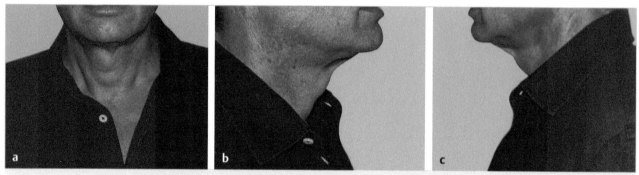

Fig. 16.11 Case 3. Postoperative picture (**a**) frontal view (**b**) right lateral view (**c**) left lateral view.

- Device Facetite: Power 10 W; cut off temperature 38°C; total energy delivered 1, 5 KJ.
- Total energy: 9, 5 KJ.
- Surgical time: 55 minutes.

Aspiration: 10 cc of Fat Results

Improvement of the cervicomental angle, better definition of jawline. Obvious skin tightening of the neck, but still some laxity. The patient was very pleased.

References

[1] Keramidas E, Rodopoulou S. Radiofrequency-assisted liposuction for neck and lower face adipodermal remodeling and contouring. Plast Reconstr Surg Glob Open 2016;4(8):e850

[2] Irvine Duncan D. Nonexcisional tissue tightening: creating skin surface area reduction during abdominal liposuction by adding radiofrequency heating. Aesthet Surg J 2013;33(8):1154–1166

[3] Theodorou SJ, Paresi RJ, Chia CT. Radiofrequency-assisted liposuction device for body contouring: 97 patients under local anesthesia. Aesthetic Plast Surg 2012;36(4):767–779

[4] Hurwitz D, Smith D. Treatment of overweight patients by RFAL for aesthetic reshaping and Skin tightening Aesthetic Plast Surg 2012;36:62–71

[5] Mulholland RS, Kreindel M, FACETITE: subdermal radiofrequency skin tightening and face contouring

[6] Paul M, Mulholland RS. A new approach for adipose tissue treatment and body contouring using radiofrequency-assisted liposuction. Aesthetic Plast Surg 2009;33(5):687–694

[7] Baker DC. Lateral SMASectomy, plication and short scar facelifts: indications and techniques. Clin Plast Surg 2008;35(4):533–550, vi

[8] Paul M, Blugerman G, Kreindel M, Mulholland RS. Three-dimensional radiofrequency tissue tightening: a proposed mechanism and applications for body contouring. Aesthetic Plast Surg 2011;35(1):87–95

[9] Ahn DH, Mulholland RS, Duncan D, et al. Non-excisional face and neck tightening using a novel subdermal radiofrequency thermo-coagulative device. J Cosmet Dermatol Sci Appl 2011;1:8845–8851

[10] Divaris M, Boisnic S, Brachet M, et al. A clinical and histological study of radiofrequency-assistedliposuction (RFAL) mediated skin tightening and cellulite improvement. J Cosmet Dermatol Sci Appl 2011;1:36–42

[11] Waldman A, Comparison of Treatment Uniformity of Laser Assisted Liposuction (LAL) and Radiofrequency-Assisted Liposuction (RFAL): Scientific Report (PhD), Israel

[12] Alexiades-Armenakas M. Combination laser-assisted liposuction and minimally invasive skin tightening with temperature feedback for treatment of the submentum and neck. Dermatol Surg 2012;38(6):871–881

[13] Ellenbogen R, Karlin JV. Visual criteria for success in restoring the youthful neck. Plast Reconstr Surg 1980;66(6):826–837

[14] Giampapa V, Bitzos I, Ramirez O, Granick M. Suture suspension platysmaplasty for neck rejuvenation revisited: technical fine points for improving outcomes. Aesthetic Plast Surg 2005;29(5):341–350, discussion 351–352

17 Neck Liposuction: The Classic Technique

Steven M. Levine

Abstract

Improving the neck and jawline contour can be accomplished through several ways. As we age, we can develop excess fat in our neck, our neck structures descend, and the skin and muscles become lax. Neck liposuction treats only the excess fat in the neck. However, it has been noted by many surgeons over many decades that removal of subcutaneous neck fat results in not only improved shape from the diminished fat, but also in neck skin tightening. To some surprise, this remains true in older people as well as younger people. Here we provide details into our preferred methods that take advantage of precise execution of classic tumescent liposuction techniques to improve the neck and jawline contour.

Keywords: Liposuction, neck liposuction, classic liposuction, suction lipectomy, neck

---

Key Points

- Neck liposuction is a powerful technique that can enhance the jawline and restore a youthful contour to the neck.

17.1 Patient Evaluation

Several attributes of the neck require examination to accurately assess its aging. These include the notation of excess skin, quality of skin elasticity, subcutaneous fat, subplatysmal fat, presence of platysma bands, prominent submandibular glands, and finally the architecture of the mandible, most notably the position of the pogonion.

When considering non-excisional procedures, skin quality is perhaps the most important factor. There is no specific test that will allow the surgeon to judge the extent of skin retraction (or tightening) that can be achieved from any particular non-excisional procedure. We caution relying on industry photos or paid speakers to set expectations. Rather, the surgeon needs to perform these procedures, in the setting of full disclosure that extent of skin tightening is unpredictable and that if not enough tightening is seen to meet the patient's desires, an excisional procedure may be necessary. The authors have been very pleased with patient satisfaction following "original" neck liposuction and in over 1000 patients treated, very few have desired an immediate excisional procedure. However, it is common for these patients to return years later for more extensive neck rejuvenation.

17.2 Preoperative Planning and Preparation

The primary objective of the preoperative plans is to resolve the patients' goals with their anatomy. Liposuction is capable of significantly reducing subcutaneous fat and creates a range skin retraction from modest to impressive by undermining and redraping the skin.

Younger patients typically have more elasticity to their skin; however, we have observed excellent results in patients in the 50s, 60s, and early 70s.

Subcutaneous fat can be distinguished from subplatysmal fat by palpating the submental or submandibular regions and asking the patient to swallow. Fat that does not "pull away" is usually subcutaneous.

17.3 Surgical Technique

17.3.1 Skin Preparation

The skin is cleaned with either betadine or chlorhexidine prior to the operation.

17.3.2 Anesthesia

Neck liposuction can be performed under local anesthesia. The authors generally use monitored anesthesia care (MAC) for these cases.

All patient's necks are infiltrated with 0.5% lidocaine with 1:400,000 epinephrine. Between 50 and 200 cc are infiltrated using a long 22 g spinal needle to administer the solution in the subcutaneous plane. Usually lipoaspirate is approximately 1:1 with infiltration.

17.3.3 Marking

All patients are marked while sitting up. The mandibular border is always marked to avoid unintentional suction of the lower face. The area to be liposuctioned varies between patients but the extent of the undermining with the cannula is always wider than the submentum, the area with the greatest concentration of fat.

17.3.4 Patient Positioning

During the surgery, the patient is laid supine with a roll beneath their shoulders to help extend the neck. The head is ideally positioned just above the most cranial portion of the table. The surgeon is standing at the head and uses his or her non-dominant hand on the mandible to extend the neck.

17.3.5 Technique

A stab incision is always made in the submental crease. Sharp scissors are used to dissect into the subcutaneous plane before using a Mercedes cannula for liposuction. This incision heals well and it is better to make the incision wider than the width of the cannula in order to avoid a friction burn on the skin.

Our workhorse cannulas are 1.8 mm and 2.4 mm. A 1.8 mm cannula is for refinement or to suction individual neck rolls via a separate lateral stab incision so that liposuction can be carried out in a transverse direction.

During the procedure, when necessary, an assistant is used to help maintain appropriate countertraction. A thin layer of fat is maintained beneath the dermis to avoid the appearance of the skin adhering to muscle and avoid damage to the subdermal plexus. To evenly remove fat but maintain a layer below the dermis, the cannula must be inserted at a level a few millimeters below the dermis and then it must constantly be moving in a fan-shaped trajectory (▶ Fig. 17.1). The surgeon should reposition the cannula at various places within the access incision (▶ Fig. 17.2). Palpation of the flap along with audible

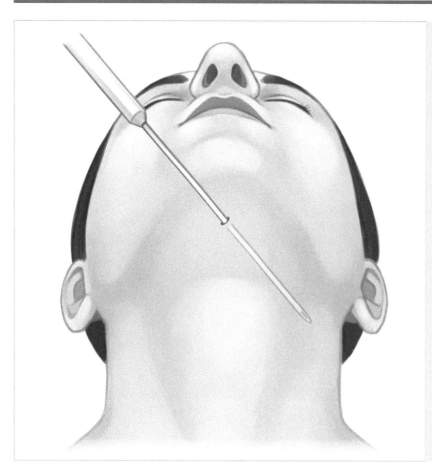

Fig. 17.1 Cannula excursion with a single submental access point.

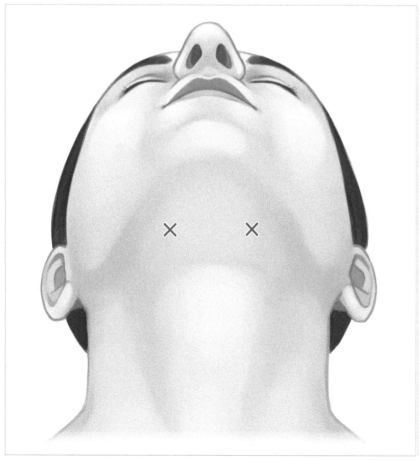

Fig. 17.2 Cannula excursion with 2 paramedian access points.

cues reflecting an "emptying" of the fat compartment are used to determine the endpoint of the liposuction.

When needed, access incisions behind the earlobes can be used to achieve a separate vector sculpting the angle of the mandible and add another vector to sculpt the neck.

At the end of the surgery, a simple stitch is used to close the submental incision. The retrolobular access points are usually left open for drainage (▶ Fig. 17.3).

17.3.6 Ancillary Procedures

In favor of direct neck defatting with scissors, neck liposuction is frequently performed alongside traditional face and necklifts.

However, there is probably no surgical procedure that compliments neck liposuction more than the placement of a chin implant. This procedure can be performed through the same submental incision and adds virtually no recovery time. The key to this procedure is to dissect a subperiosteal pocket that is the same size or slightly smaller than the actual chin implant. When this is well-executed, no fixation of the implant is required.

17.3.7 Postoperative Care

Immediately after surgery, a xeroform gauze is laid over the neck followed by a bulky dressing of unwrapped gauze and ABD pads. A Surgiflex net is placed over this bulky dressing and kept on for 24–48 hours. After this dressing is removed, patients are given soft cervical collars to prevent them from excessive turning of the heads to allow the skin flap to adhere without shearing forces.

17.3.8 Healing

Patients usually feel fine the next day. The jaw may be tender and the undermined skin is temporarily numb. Mild to moderate edema and ecchymosis is expected after surgery and usually subsides enough within 3–5 days to allow for normal social interaction. It is rare for a patient to require more than over the counter pain medication.

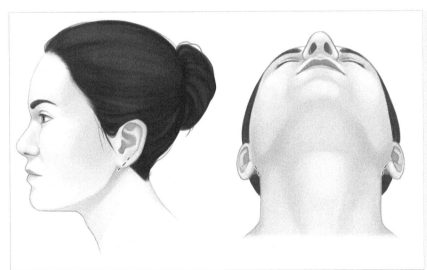

Fig. 17.3 Benefits of retroauricular access points.

17.4 Results and Outcomes

Dramatic results are usually observed at the time of dressing removal, however healing continues for a year.

17.5 Problems and Complications

Complications requiring surgical intervention are exceedingly rare. Seromas and hematomas are the most likely complications; however, appropriate compression dressing should mitigate that risk. The major complication concerns relate to oversuctioning. Specifically if a layer of fat is not preserved on the skin flap, dermal injury can occur yielding two virtually uncorrectable consequences. These include dermal scarring that appears similar to platysmal bands and skeletonization of neck, which tends to make patients look older, not more youthful. However, given liposuction is a closed procedure, it is can be difficult to assess the quantity of fat remaining on the skin flap. For this reason, it is always better to leave excess fat than remove too much. It is far better to have to return to the OR to remove a few more milliliters of fat than be forced to deal with the alternative.

18 Radiofrequency-Assisted Liposuction for Arm Contouring

Spero J. Theodorou, Christopher T. Chia, and Stelios C. Wilson

Abstract

Arm contouring has traditionally been addressed with liposuction alone or with skin excision procedures. More specifically, liposuction is offered to individuals with mild skin laxity and good skin quality while all others are considered candidates for brachioplasty. Given the scar burden that accompanies brachioplasty, may individuals with moderate or severe skin laxity defer surgery leaving a relatively large treatment gap. In this chapter, we offer our treatment algorithm for patients based on skin laxity and skin quality. Through the addition of radiofrequency-assisted liposuction (RFAL), we are able to treat patients with excess fat and moderate to severe skin laxity without necessarily committing these patients to the scar burden of traditional brachioplasty. To that end, we offer our technique to provide safe and reproducible results using this technology. RFAL is a powerful tool for thermal contraction of the soft tissues in properly selected cases.

Keywords: Arm contouring, body contouring, brachioplasty, liposuction, radiofrequency, radiofrequency-assisted liposuction, RFAL

Contouring of the arms has always posed a distinct challenge to plastic surgeons due to the dependent nature of the underlying skin and its non-adherence to the underlying structures. Although brachioplasty has been an effective procedure for patients with massive weight loss and severe laxity it entails a long unsightly scar that often heals poorly. The reason being that these wounds are subject to a combination of gravity-induced tension, weighted flap design, and the nature of non-adherence of the area. The number of patients asking for a solution to this deformity far supersedes the number of patients settling for a brachioplasty operation. Even though there have been classifications of arm deformities in the past (there have never really been clear treatment pathways other than brachioplasty offered for advanced ptosis).[1,2] As such, arm contouring is defined to an extent by a treatment gap in our existing armamentarium of solutions offered to patients.

Technology-based solutions have been offered up in the past. Older treatment modalities such as ultrasound-assisted liposuction and superficial subdermal liposuction have been reported to have some effect on skin retraction in this area.[3] However, the first comes with questionable results and the second carries significant risks for contour deformities. Radiofrequency-assisted liposuction presents a novel approach to arm contouring with reproducible results.[4] This is achieved via the generated electromagnetic energy of a bipolar device designed to heat the soft tissues and cause contraction and collagen formation.

18.1 Anatomical RFAL Arm Landmarks

The patient is marked in the standing position with his or her arms to the side touching the lateral thighs. This is a perfect position to mark the deltoid fat pad (DFP) and its projection as well as the fat overlying the triceps. The arm is then positioned with the elbow flexed at 90 degrees in order to allow proper examination of the underlying soft tissues that are inferior to the bicipital groove. The bicipital groove is then marked (▶Fig. 18.1).

18.2 No Man's Land

The area between the bicipital groove and the DFP border is outlined as "no man's land". This area, as the name implies, is not treated. It carries significant treatment risk due to the underlying neurovascular structures (▶Fig. 18.2).

18.3 Zone 1 and Zone 2

The dependent portion of the arm is further subdivided into two treatment zones. The proximal one third "zone 1" and the distal one third "zone 2". Zone 1 typically contains more fat and contributes to the majority of the laxity seen in most cases that require arm contouring. This zone in turn will be the recipient of the majority of the RF energy (▶Fig. 18.3).

18.4 Deltoid Fat Pad

The DFP has often been overlooked in arm contouring. It not only has medical ramifications (as in inoculation injections) but also aesthetic implications. The more lateral projection of the DFP the more disconcerting it tends to be for female patients. They present with the common complaint of being too "wide" accompanied by the feelings of personal embarrassment when wearing short sleeve shirts or dresses. We call this the "linebacker" look. Modern day aesthetics of the arm beckon for a more sculpted toned appearance for both men and women. The treatment of the DFP is critical in this respect as it typically translates into high patient satisfaction[5] (▶Fig. 18.4).

18.4.1 Deltoid Fat Pad Marking

A longitudinal line is drawn along the length of the arm starting at the acromion of the scapula intersecting the deltoid muscle insertion. A transverse

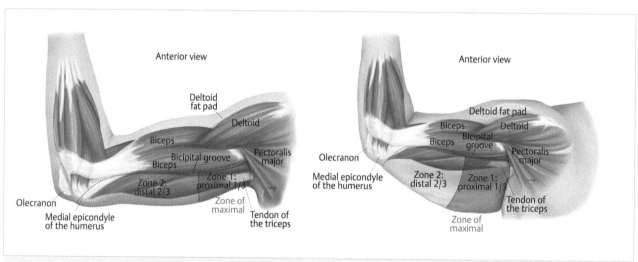

Fig. 18.1 Anatomical radiofrequency-assisted liposuction (RFAL) arm landmarks.

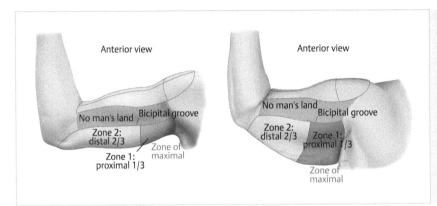

Fig. 18.2 No man's land.

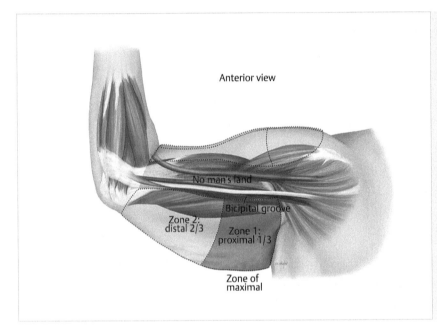

Fig. 18.3 Zone 1 and zone 2.

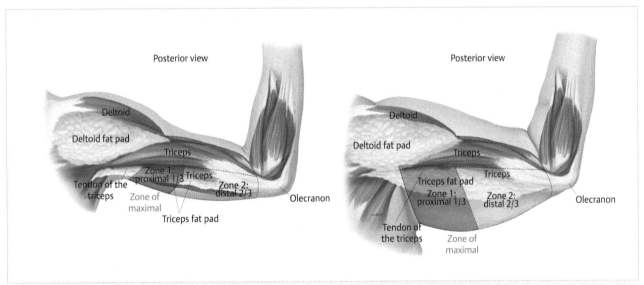

Fig. 18.4 Deltoid fat pad.
Fat pad thickness: Women 11.7 mm, men 8.3 mm.
Skinfold thickness: Women 34.6 mm, men 17.2 mm.

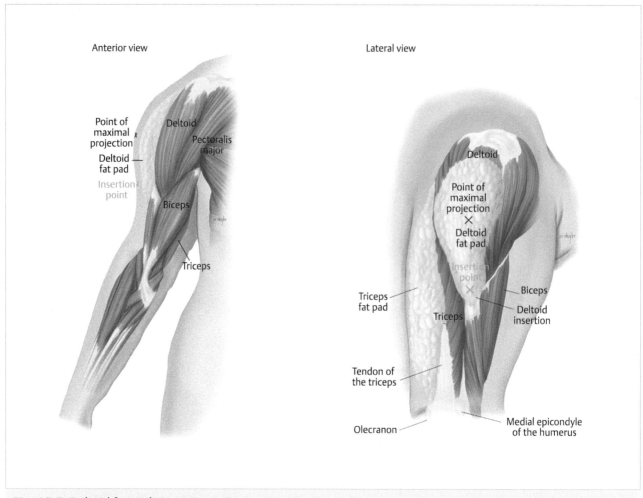

Fig. 18.5 Deltoid fat pad—insertion point.

line intersecting the longitudinal one marks the point of maximal projection. The access point is marked at approximately 3 cm distal to this point at the junction of the deltoid muscle insertion and the biceps. The natural shadow cast by the confluence of these two muscles tends to be less conspicuous of a scar (▶Fig. 18.5).

18.5 Triceps Fat Pad Marking and Treatment Parameters

The triceps midline meridian (TMM) line is defined by a longitudinal line dividing the triceps fad pad into lateral and medial treatment zones. A large amount of RF energy is deposited along this TMM line in order to facilitate contraction and tissue recruitment towards it. This acts as an internal "seam". The analogy being the excess fabric gathered and tailored in a suit (▶Fig. 18.6). Brachioplasty incisions act in a similar fashion when treating excess tissue in the arms. The difference with RFAL is that the "seam" or "incision scar" is internal in RFAL treated arms cases and hence not visible.[6]

The above methodology addresses RF energy distribution and tissue tightening. However, in order to complete the operation, arm contouring by SAL needs to follow. The arm is a cylinder-like structure and needs to be treated in

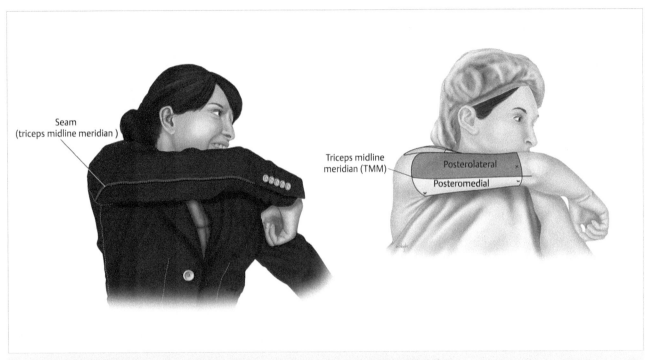

Fig. 18.6 The concept of the internal seam—triceps midline meridian (TMM).

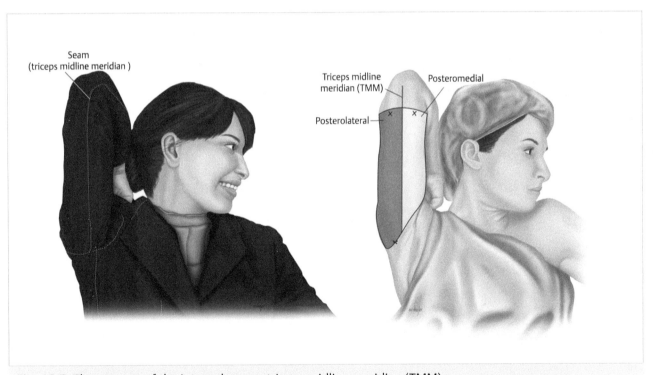

Fig. 18.7 The concept of the internal seam—triceps midline meridian (TMM).

a 3D way for optimal results (▶Fig. 18.7). In order to achieve this "gathering" of tissue along the TMM line and creating the aforementioned internal seam the operator has to perform liposuction of the arm in a 270-degree fashion (▶Fig. 18.8). This will result in discontinuous undermining of the soft

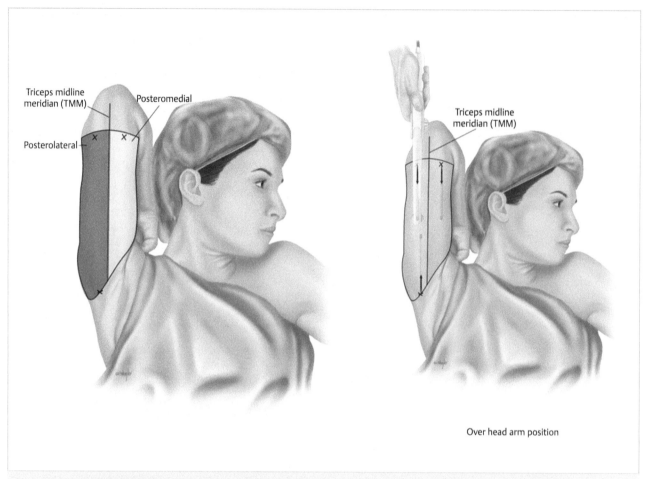

Fig. 18.8 RFAL TMM application. RFAL, radiofrequency-assisted liposuction; TMM, triceps midline meridian.

tissue envelop thus allowing for proper release and re-draping of the skin. The benefit of this approach will be the reduction in the circumference of the arm with simultaneous tightening of the preoperative laxity (▶Fig. 18.9).

18.6 RFAL Arm Candidate Selection

We devised a classification that is the first to provide treatment solutions for arm contouring taking into consideration: degree of laxity and skin quality.[7] As such we have defined the following parameters:
- **Arm skin laxity (ASL):** Distance measured between the most dependent point of the skin of the arm; point of maximal dependency (PMD) in the 90 batwing position and the corresponding perpendicular point on the bicipital groove. The ASL ranges from mild (less than 5 cm), moderate (5–10 cm) to severe (more than 10 cm) (▶Fig. 18.10).
- **Arm skin quality (ASQ):** Quality of skin evaluated by pinch and subjective assessment for dermal thickness, tone, presence or absence of striae and Fitzpatrick skin type. It is classified as good (good skin turgor, no striae, and an absence of fine wrinkling) or poor (moderate to poor skin turgor, presence of striae and fine wrinkles).

All arms are evaluated for presence or absence of fat and FSN. These two parameters as well as the thickness of the dermis are the three most important factors that affect contraction with RFAL.
▶Table 18.1 is a guide to energy based arm contouring.

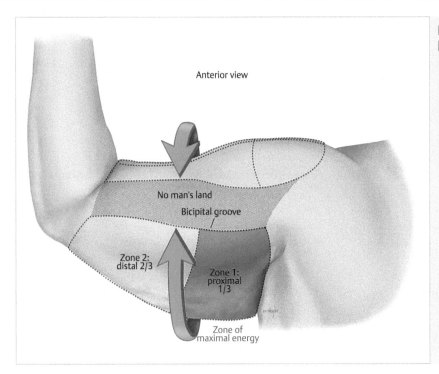

Fig. 18.9 Circumferential liposuction 270°.

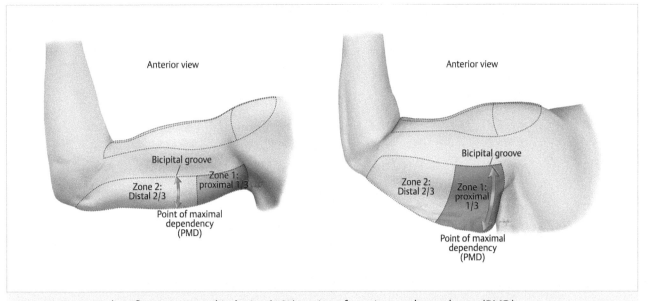

Fig. 18.10 Arm classification—arm skin laxity (ASL): point of maximum dependency (PMD).

Table 18.1 Arm classification

	ASL	ASQ	Adiposity	Treatment
Type I	Mild	Good	-	Not RFAL candidate
Type II	Moderate	Good	+	SAL/LAL
Type III	Moderate	Poor	+	RFAL
Type IV	Severe	Good	+	RFAL
Type V	Severe	Poor	+	RFAL+ staged skin excision
Type VI	Severe	Poor	-	Brachioplasty

Abbreviations: ASL, arm skin laxity; ASQ, arm skin quality; LAL, laser-assisted liposuction; RFAL, radiofrequency-assisted liposuction; SAL, suction-assisted liposuction.

18.7 Radiofrequency Application

The RFAL external probe is set at 38–40°C. The internal probe is set at 65°C. The RF device is preset at 20 W and this cannot be modified for safety purposes. The depth wheel is set to 3–4 cm depending on the thickness of the tissue treated. Access puncture incisions are made with a 14 gauge needle at the elbow, axilla, and deltoid. Bacitracin ointment is used liberally to minimize friction at the access points. Tumescent solution of 400 mg of lidocaine (0.04%) and 1 mL of 1:1000 concentration per liter normal saline is inserted into the area to be treated. If the procedure is carried under local anesthesia (authors' preference) the lidocaine amount is increased to 1000 mg per 1 L of normal saline (▶ Fig. 18.11).

Sterile ultrasound gel is applied to the surface of the skin in order to decrease impedance between the probes. The RF handpiece is then inserted through the access port in the elbow. The movement of the handpiece is identical to liposuction albeit much slower. Utilizing the axillary and elbow incisions in alternate motion the energy is applied until the target temperature is reached. This manifests itself as an audible bell emanating from the machine. Care must be taken to focus the energy on the TMM and to spend a minimum of 1–3 minutes to recreate the internal seam. As the heating progresses more superficially the distance between the two electrodes–calipers is closed. This in effect results in lesser tissue being treated as we get closer to the undersurface of the dermis. The endpoint is the target temperature of 38–42°C.

The contouring part of the operation is then started after removal of the RF handpiece. This is performed by using a 4–0 mm Double Mercedes PAL Microaire (Charlottesville, VA) cannula followed by a 3–0 mm Double Mercedes for finer more superficial contouring (▶ Fig. 18.12). Once this is complete the access incisions are closed with 5–0 nylon and a garment is applied. For fat volume aspirations of more than 800 cc–1 lt, a drain is recommended. This is removed on average after 2–3 days. Arm garment compression is recommended for 4–6 weeks postoperatively.

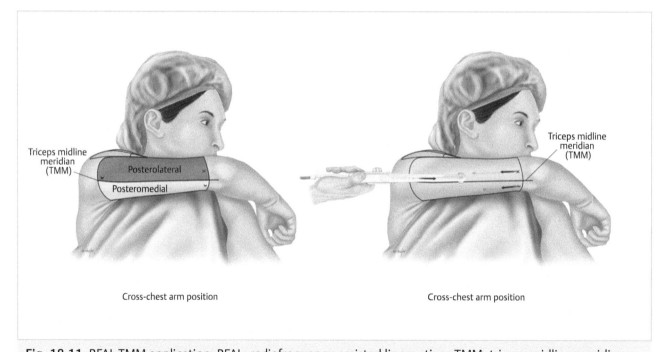

Fig. 18.11 RFAL TMM application. RFAL, radiofrequency-assisted liposuction; TMM, triceps midline meridian.

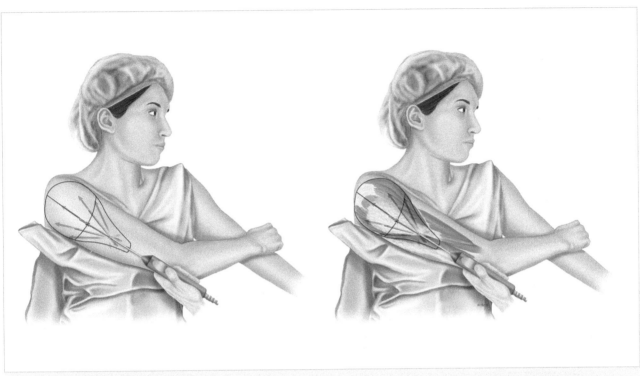

Fig. 18.12 Deltoid fat pad—SAL 3 mm mercedes.

18.8 Conclusion

Patients with excess fat and moderate to severe laxity no longer have to be automatically considered brachioplasty candidates. They now have options. RFAL mediated thermal contraction of the soft tissue in properly selected cases can result in reproducible results with high patient satisfaction levels.[8] Striving to produce arm contouring results that are free of long incisions and unsightly scars should be every plastic surgeon's goal in the future. RFAL allows us to get closer to that goal.

References

[1] El Khatib HA. Classification of brachial ptosis: strategy for treatment. Plast Reconstr Surg 2007; 119(4):1337–1342

[2] Appelt EA, Janis JE, Rohrich RJ. An algorithmic approach to upper arm contouring. Plast Reconstr Surg 2006; 118(1):237–246

[3] Gasperoni C, Gasperoni P. Subdermal liposuction: long-term experience. Clin Plast Surg 2006; 33(1):63–73, vi

[4] Duncan DI. Improving outcomes in upper arm liposuction: adding radiofrequency-assisted liposuction to induce skin contraction. Aesthet Surg J 2012; 32(1):84–95

[5] Theodorou SJ, Paresi RJ, Chia CT. Radiofrequency-assisted liposuction device for body contouring: 97 patients under local anesthesia. Aesthetic Plastic Surgery

[6] Theodorou S, Chia C. Radiofrequency-assisted liposuction for arm contouring: technique under local anesthesia. Plast Reconstr Surg Glob Open 2013; 1(5):e37

[7] Chia CT, Theodorou SJ, Hoyos AE, Pitman GH. Radiofrequency-assisted liposuction compared with aggressive superficial, subdermal liposuction of the arms: a bilateral quantitative comparison. Plast Reconstr Surg Glob Open 2015; 3(7):e459

[8] Chia CT, Neinstein RM, Theodorou SJ. Evidence-based medicine: liposuction MOC-CME. Plast Reconstr Surg 2017; 139:267e

19 FaceTite: Procedure Technique

P. Paolo Rovatti

Abstract

Tissue tightening is one of the most common demands in aesthetic surgery worldwide and the primary purpose of an energy device is to provide an improvement of skin quality.

Skin laxity, with or without fat, of the lower third of the face is one of the main signs of an aging face.

Skin tightening procedures are among the most interesting innovations in the growing market of energy devices for a youthful face. We've reviewed our experience in the last six years with a bipolar radiofrequency (RF) energy device called FaceTite, which gave us a satisfactory result in terms of no-excisional procedure and long-lasting effectiveness.

Goals of this surgery are: local anesthesia technique, reduced procedure time, minimal downtime, great patient acceptance, and satisfying long-lasting results.

Many safety controls were introduced in order to improve the reliability of this device, and thanks to recent refinements the learning curve for this instrument has been shortened significantly. Combining synchronously this technique with fractional bipolar RF (Morpheus8) to improve "in and out" thermal stimulation in dermis, we can produce a marvelous change of the skin.

In conclusion, we can assert that this technology has shown diverse advantages, also thanks to the recent improvements in safety control and can thus be a powerful tool for surgeons and a reliable choice for patients.

Keywords: Radiofrequency, skin tightening, FaceTite, noninvasive lifting, jawline ptosis, neck laxity

Radiofrequency is a relatively young technique that allows energy to be applied to the tissues in a bipolar manner, inside as coagulative energy and externally as cutaneous heating. This dual approach makes it possible to obtain a contraction of the fibrous septa and at the same time a cutaneous retraction.[1]

RF has been widely used in association with traditional liposuction, thanks to its tissue contraction action, which allows to carry out the procedure even in the presence of tissue laxity. This feature led in recent years to the recognition of RF as the method to prefer in cases of laxity of the region of the mandibular edge and neck, with or without adipose excess tissue.

Both male and female patients may be treated with cutaneous laxity of the mandibular border, the submental region, and the neck with or without fat accumulation. The preoperative evaluation is performed according to the Merz scales for neck and mandibular line and patients with a neck grade from 1 to 4 and a jawline grade from 1 to are considered suitable for treatment. The treatment of patient with higher degrees of tissue failure unfortunately results in partial and often unsatisfactory results and therefore they are considered a contra-indication related to the procedure.

It should also be considered that the presence of significant skin failure and a loss of adipose volume (1–2 grade Carruthers scale) with a high degree of photo and chronoaging (III–IV type in Glogau scale), represents a further contraindication to the treatment.

FaceTite is the device that belongs to the Body Tite equipment (Invasix Ltd, Israel), which is used for the treatment of the face and neck. This handpiece transmits a thermal effect to the adipose tissue determining a coagulation.

The heat then radiates progressively towards the skin, crossing the derma to full-thickness, thus promoting the skin tightening effect (▶Fig. 19.1). The procedure is usually performed with subcutaneous infiltrative anesthesia (wet technique) using 20 mL of lidocaine 200 mg/10 mL + 60 cc of saline solution + 0.5 mL of epinephrine 1:1000.[2]

The surgical treatment consists of introducing the internal probe of the handpiece through a small hole made with a 16 G needle, which must maintain a depth level between 5 and 8 mm (▶Fig. 19.2). The correct alignment of

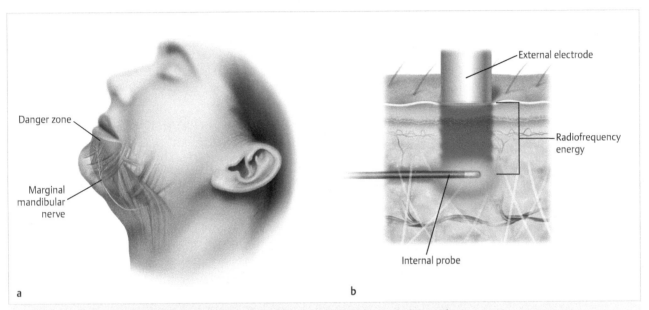

Danger zone

Marginal mandibular nerve

External electrode

Radiofrequency energy

Internal probe

a

b

Fig. 19.1 (a) Area to be treated carefully. (b) Safe area below internal electrode.

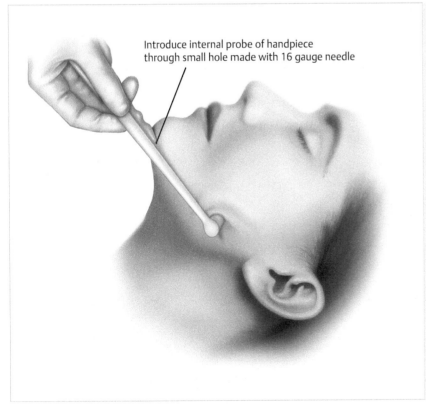

Introduce internal probe of handpiece through small hole made with 16 gauge needle

Fig. 19.2 Treatment modality.

the two internal and external electrodes grants uniform heating of the tissue in its entire thickness. Radiofrequency energy is transmitted better through the vertical fibrous septa network (FSN) that is a path of least resistance and is parallel to the RF delivered.[3] RF[4] energy is transmitted preferentially in vertical FSN vs. horizontal layers which are perpendicular to the RF[5,6] and this leads to more tightening effects on the fat tissue.[7] The range of the internal temperature must remain between 65 and 70°C and allows the coagulation and contraction of the septa within the adipose tissue in a three-dimensional manner; on the cutaneous level the cut-off must remain within 38 and 40°C with consequent lower heat density, but with an effective skin tightening effect.

The handpiece is equipped with two sensors (internal and external) that control the subcutaneous and skin temperature until the energy supply is interrupted when the set parameters are reached. The delivery of the RF is automatically stopped also when the distance between the two electrodes increases or decreases too much: for example, if the internal probe is too superficial or when treating areas with curvatures. The device is also equipped with an impedance control system, which permits radiofrequency to be delivered only when the external handpiece is in full contact with the skin. As the subdermal temperature increases, the impedance is reduced, but if this happens too quickly, FaceTite stops automatically, thereby preventing skin burns.[8] This automatic control system allows treatment of surface fat without excessive risk of thermal damage. Radiofrequency delivers energy only between the cannula and the external electrode, preventing energy from being distributed below the cannula itself, then into the subfascial districts, hence avoiding harmful effects on vessel and nerves.

The handpiece is introduced through three holes: one in the submental region and two submandibular ones in the inferior-lateral margin of the DAO (LMF entry). These latter access points are used to treat the area above the mandibular edge by directing the handpiece towards the ear and then the area below the mandibular edge, in the lateral-cervical region.

From the submental access we proceed then to carry out the treatment of the interplatismatic region, moving the handpiece in caudo-cranial direction with fan-like technique.

Radiofrequency must be delivered with a retrograde movement in the district to be treated. In the area of the mandibular edge the treatment must be performed above and below the edge. The first passage is carried out slowly, stopping for about 1 second, and no more, every 1–2 cm to determine the decrease in tissue thickness, thanks to the vertical contraction of the connective septa. During this phase it will be easy to hear a crackle (popping sound) which is a sign of the coagulative necrosis of the superficial fatty tissue, immediately subdermal. The next passage, on the other hand, occurs with a slow but continuous movement in the previously tunneled tissue until the cut-off is reached.

The neck is conventionally divided into 3 parts: the interplatismatic region is reached through the submental access, while the two lateral areas through the submandibular accesses (▶ Fig. 19.3). The treatment of the neck requires the use of the FaceTite handpiece with continuous retrograde technique until the cut-off is reached. The energy delivered in the region of the mandibular edge is 1.5–2.5 kJ per side, while in the neck is about 3–6 kJ of total energy.

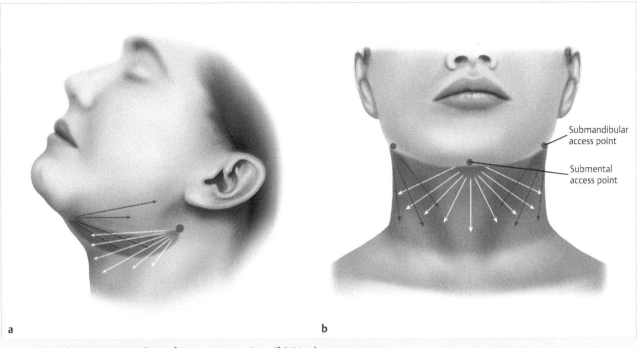

Fig. 19.3 **(a)** Treatment lines from entry point. **(b)** Neck treatment.

Liposuction before radiofrequency is never performed; if the fat excess in the submental region is particularly evident (fat plication greater than 1.5 cm), at the end of the procedure an aspiration of the liquefied fat with microcannula can be carried out, not more than 2 cc.

Patient selection should include moderate to medium-high ptosis of both the jawline and neck. Recent great weight loss may cause unsatisfactory results and therefore it is really important to wait for the patient to return in acceptable metabolic balance.

Absolute contraindications are patients with pacemaker, silicone or permanent fillers in the areas to be treated, while no contraindications should be considered with previous treatments in the involved areas (threadlift, previous facelift, fillers HA and CaHA). We found relative contraindications treating previous laserlipo procedures.

To maximize the results, this procedure can be combined with the transdermal fractional radiofrequency (Morpheus8) which, in the same session, can further improve skin tightening.

Using the local anesthesia previously done, the transdermal device with 24 needles is applied on the skin overlapping 30/40% on all neck areas reaching a result after two/three treatment (each apart 45 days) with a GAIS improvement scale of 74% by the patient (▶ Fig. 19.4).[5,6,7,9,10,11,12,13,14,15,16]

The procedure now is safer thanks to the new device cut-off control. The internal sensor cut-off precludes the fat from liquefying and creating possible necrosis thus reducing the possible related complications. No permanent thermal-related injuries were observed among our patients. Only a few neuropraxias of the mental nerve (four cases) were pointed out, each one pharmacologically resolved after few months.

Skin burns due to excessively superficial treatment resolved spontaneously without scarring. Persistent swelling (more than two months) was found in only few cases and was successfully resolved with manual lymphatic drainage. In conclusion, we can affirm that in this procedure, the relationship between minimal side effects and good results seems to be favorable.

19.1 Patient Cases

See ▶ Fig. 19.5, ▶ Fig. 19.6, ▶ Fig. 19.7, and ▶ Fig. 19.8.

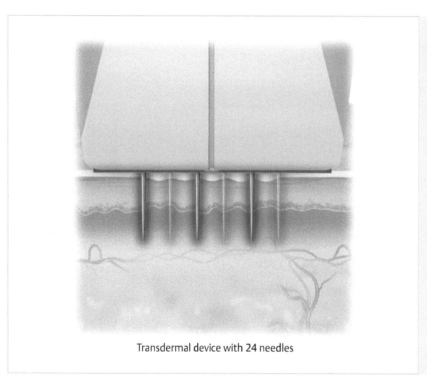

Transdermal device with 24 needles

Fig. 19.4 Fractional transdermal heating.

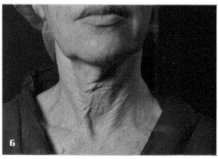
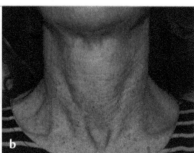

Fig. 19.5 (a) Preoperative. Woman 65 y Baker type 4. (b) 1 year postoperative: 1 FaceTite surgery 8 K/J tot + 3 Fractora neck treatment 45 W.

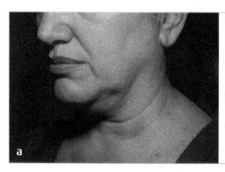
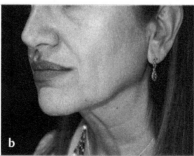

Fig. 19.6 (a) Preoperative. Lateral view, 56 y Baker type 3. (b) Postoperative. 56 y. 2 years postoperative one FaceTite treatment 10 K/J tot after 22 kg weight loss result stable.

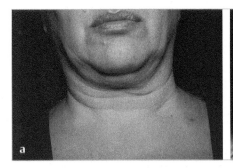
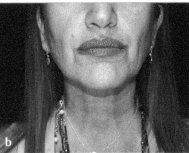

Fig. 19.7 **(a)** Preoperative. Front view, 56 y Baker type 3. **(b)** Postoperative. After 24 months, 22 kg weight loss one FaceTite treatment 10 K/J tot.

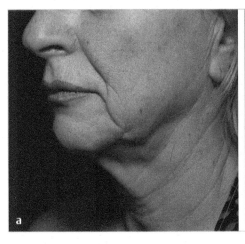
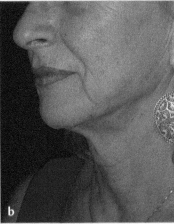

Fig. 19.8 **(a)** Preoperative. 58 7 Baker type 4 face lift candidate, neck laxity. **(b)** 4 months postoperative, one FaceTite 8.5 K/J two fractora treatment 35 W.

References

[1] Jimenez Lozano JN, Vacas-Jacques P, Anderson RR, Franco W. Effect of fibrous septa in radiofrequency heating of cutaneous and subcutaneous tissues: computational study. Lasers Surg Med 2013;45(5):326–338

[2] Theodorou S, Chia C. Radiofrequency-assisted liposuction for arm contouring: technique under local anesthesia. Plast Reconstr Surg Glob Open 2013;1(5):e37

[3] Duncan DI. Nonexcisional tissue tightening: creating skin surface area reduction during abdominal liposuction by adding radiofrequency heating. Aesthet Surg J 2014;33:1154–1166

[4] DiBernardo BE. Randomized, blinded split abdomen study evaluating skin shrinkage and skin tightening in laser-assisted liposuction versus liposuction control. Aesthet Surg J 2010;30(4):593–602

[5] Paul M, Blugerman G, Kreindel M, Mulholland RS. Three-dimensional radiofrequency tissue tightening: a proposed mechanism and applications for body contouring. Aesthetic Plast Surg 2011;35(1):87–95

[6] Paul M, Mulholland RS. A new approach for adipose tissue treatment and body contouring using radiofrequency-assisted liposuction. Aesthetic Plast Surg 2009;33(5):687–694

[7] Treatment of Décolletage Photoaging with Fractional Microneedling Radiofrequency. Lyons A, Roy J, Herrmann J, Chipps L. J Drugs Dermatol 2018;17(1):74–76

[8] Alexiades-Armenakas M. Combination laser-assisted liposuction and minimally invasive skin tightening with temperature feedback for treatment of the submentum and neck. Dermatol Surg 2012;38(6):871–881

[9] Thanasarnaksorn W, Siramangkhalanon V, Duncan DI, Belenky I. Fractional ablative and nonablative radiofrequency for skin resurfacing and rejuvenation of Thai patients. J Cosmet Dermatol 2018;17(2):184–192

[10] Theodorou SJ, Paresi RJ, Chia CT. Radiofrequency-assisted liposuction device for body contouring: 97 patients under local anesthesia. Aesthetic Plast Surg 2012;36(4):767–779

[11] Mulholland RS. Nonexcisional, minimally invasive rejuvenation of the neck. Clin Plast Surg 2014;41(1):11–31

[12] Ahn DH, Mulholland RS, Duncan D, Paul M. Non-excisional face and neck tightening using a novel subdermal radiofrequency thermo-coagulative device. J Cosmet Dermatol Sci Appl 2011;1:8845–8851

[13] Waldman A. Comparison of treatment uniformity of laser assisted liposuction (LAL) and radiofrequency-assisted liposuction (RFAL): scientific report (PhD). Israel

[14] Blugerman G, Schavelzon D, Paul MD. A safety and feasibility study of a novel radiofrequency-assisted liposuction technique. Plast Reconstr Surg 2010;125(3):998–1006

[15] Friedman DJ, Gilead LT. The use of hybrid radiofrequency device for the treatment of rhytides and lax skin. Dermatol Surg 2007;33(5):543–551

[16] Mulholland RS. An in depth examination of radiofrequency-assisted liposuction (RFAL). J Cosmetic Surg Medicine 2009;4(3):14–19

20 Male Gynecomastia Treatment

Alfredo Hoyos and David E. Guarin

Abstract

Gynecomastia is a very common and embarrassing male condition characterized by enlargement of the fat and glandular tissue. To understand the esthetic disruption and to make a correct diagnosis is very important to know the characteristics of the ideal shape of the anterior chest wall.

The three main gynecomastia components (skin, fat, and gland) have to be addressed in order to achieve an adequate result.

Fat grafting is crucial to get a muscular appearance. The VASER aids in facilitating the extraction, reduce bleeding, and induce skin retraction. The dense glandular tissue requires open resection.

Keywords: Gynecomastia, pectoral definition, VASER, male liposuction, high definition

The abnormal growth of breast tissue in males or gynecomastia is a benign condition in which glandular and fat tissue is misplaced. This condition can be physically and psychologically uncomfortable, negatively impacting self- confidence and body image. This condition can affect one on both sides, especially at the extremes of life. In youngsters, this condition can appear and can be as high as 60% of the population but most of the time the condition is temporal.

20.1 The Beautiful Normal: Male Pectoral Anatomy and Beauty Standards

Male anatomy in the pectoral area is simple, it is just the superficial transparency of the pectoralis muscle and surrounding musculoskeletal structures. The pectoral muscle extends from the medial half of the clavicle, the sternocostal head and the sternum up to the superior 6 costal cartilages and the aponeurosis of the external oblique and rectus sheath.

The ideal male pectoral shape has withstood time and cultural differences. The artistic male torso representation across cultures describes it as having a well-developed pectoralis major and a thin skin layer that gently exposes the anatomy beneath.

The pectorals muscle for essential aesthetics analysis can be divided into upper and lower pole, however in a more purist sense in an upper/internal pole, and a lower/external one. The division between these two sections is drawn by a line between the anterior axillary fold and the midline point crossing the lower pectoralis border (▶ Fig. 20.1).

The upper/internal pole of the muscle is the one that must have a volume enhancement to achieve visibility and the impression of a powerful muscle.

The lower/external pole is the one that beneficiate from a resection and/or volume reduction. When the pectoral area is enhanced, is important to restore the lateral and lower border of the pectoralis muscle to eliminate the "fatty" or "female" look in this area. So the straight lines of the pectoralis major insertion should be accentuated to avoid the curviness of the breast tissue.

The superficial skin anatomy must match the deep structures in a way that the lower border of the areola should align with the lower border of the

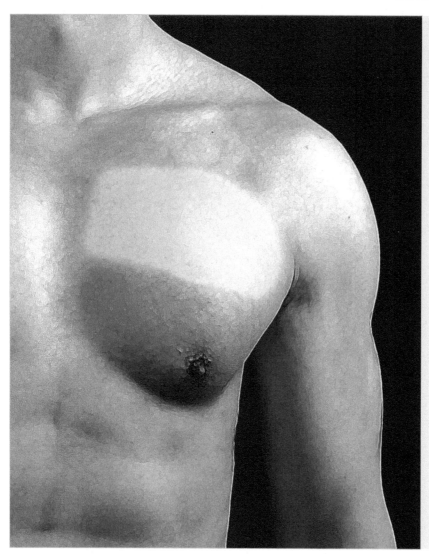

Fig. 20.1 Pectoralis major aesthetic division.

pectoralis muscle. The areola is to be placed over a vertical line between the mid clavicle and extend the lateral third. This landmark is important, because when a pectoral tuck is needed the lateral movement of the areola can fall in a non-anatomical site.

20.2 Analysis of the Male Chest Deformities: Skin versus Gland versus Fat

When approaching the patient-specific deformity all the chest components must be taken into account separately to choose the most accurate technique and by predicting how much of the skin is going to retract after the mixed approach. Many different classification scales can be found in the literature however the proposed by Rohrich in 2003 and by Cordova and Moschella in 2008 are both reasonably simple and easy to use.

The individual patient analysis must give the idea of the amount of gland, fat, and skin. This information can be translated to a classification of severity and leads to a guide to choosing the ideal method. The fat component can be extracted by means of liposuction, the glandular may need an open resection and the third component, the skin, can be managed by means of resection or a tightening technique.

20.3 Algorithm for the Surgical Options in Male Gynecomastia; Male Specific

Derived from an accurate analysis of the components of the defects and we propose a classification according to surgical choices:
• Grade 1: Liposuction alone.
• Grade 2: Liposuction and glandular excision using an omega pattern.
• Grade 3: Liposuction and glandular excision using an omega pattern: skin tightening technology such as radiofrequency.
• Grade 4: Liposuction and glandular excision using a periareolar incision for reduction.
• Grade 5: Liposuction and glandular excision, pectoral tuck using axillary incision, with or without areolar mobilization.

20.4 The Role of Fat Grafting to Enhance the Muscular Appearance and Reduce the Scar in Surgical Options

After the initial treatment, the result is an empty pectoral area that solves the female-like appearance but is far from being an ideal pectoral. The athletic patient achieves an ideal shape after expending long hours exercising by weightlifting and adequate nutrition.

This shape can also be achieved by selectively grafting the pectoral muscle upper pole and by this volume increase also reduces the amount of loose skin and the need for removal.

20.5 VASER Gynecomastia: VASER Mixed Approach to Induce Skin Retraction and Reduce Bleeding

The use of third-generation ultrasound can diminish the amount of bleeding while performing reduction of the pectoral fat. This is performed by using first infiltration 2:1 in the area and surroundings. First on the superficial layer, and later on the deep fat layer. The ultrasound is initiated on the superficial layer usually 70% in pulsed mode. Later we proceed to the deep layer in 70 to 90% in continuous mode. This allows us to emulsify fat and skeletonize the breast tissue remaining. Liposuction is performed also first on the deep layer to remove the extra fat that is hiding the muscles. The emphasis is done in the lower section of the pectoralis area. The division between these two sections is drawn by a line between the anterior axillary fold and the midline point crossing the lower pectoralis border. An extensive removal of the remaining breast tissue is performed doing liposuction with a Baker cannula (basket). If after the procedure there is this remnant breast tissue that is resilient to liposuction, we change to an open approach.

20.6 Open Access for Gynecomastic Tissue: Inverted Omega Incision

The incision is an extension of the liposuction access at the lower border of the nipple: an inverted omega following a semicircle in the lower border of nipple and two branches in a horizontal manner until meeting the areolar border. This can give an exposure of 3 to 4 cm wide, enough to perform any glandular resection through an open access. Open excision with scissors is done starting just underneath the nipple, and extending all around to remove all the remaining gland.

20.7 Complications, Prevention, and Treatment

The most expected complication is the hematoma, usually reported in open excision of the remaining gland, prevention begins by a conscious cauterization of the bleeders.

Another possible complication is related to fat grafting, can be divided into two: one due to the presence of fat cysts and second because of an infection of the area. These can be prevented by using an adequate technique and a little manipulation of the fat before insertion in fat grafting. The use of antibiotics as additive to the fat mixture can help also to prevent infections.

Suggested Readings

Barros AC, Sampaio M de CM. Gynecomastia: physiopathology, evaluation and treatment. Sao Paulo Med J 2012;130(3):187–197

Cordova A, Moschella F. Algorithm for clinical evaluation and surgical treatment of gynaecomastia. J Plast Reconstr Aesthet Surg 2008;61(1):41–49

Hoyos A, Perez M. Dynamic-definition male pectoral reshaping and enhancement in slim, athletic, obese, and gynecomastic patients through selective fat removal and grafting. Aesthetic Plast Surg 2012;36(5):1066–1077

Narula HS, Carlson HE. Gynaecomastia—pathophysiology, diagnosis and treatment. Nat Rev Endocrinol 2014;10(11):684–698

Pilanci O, Basaran K, Aydin HU, Cortuk O, Kuvat SV. Autologous fat injection into the pectoralis major as an adjunct to surgical correction of gynecomastia. Aesthet Surg J 2015;35(3):NP54–NP61

Sanchez ER, Sanchez R, Moliver C. Anatomic relationship of the pectoralis major and minor muscles: a cadaveric study. Aesthet Surg J 2014;34(2):258–263

Wong KY, Malata CM. Conventional versus ultrasound-assisted liposuction in gynaecomastia surgery: a 13-year review. J Plast Reconstr Aesthet Surg 2014;67(7):921–926

21 High Definition Body Contouring of the Abdomen

Alfredo Hoyos and David E. Guarin

Abstract

Abdominal enhancing is one of the most common concerns in the daily practice of the aesthetic surgeon. There are differences in the female and male ideal abdominal shape and are very important to understand and make a correct diagnosis. The type of abdominal definition procedure is determined by the individual body biotype. For the procedure, it is needed to adequately identify the particular anatomy paying special attention to the rectus abdominis muscle. Energy-based liposuction aids are very useful but requires an adequate infiltration and timing to avoid complications.

Keywords: Abdominal definition, body biotypes, muscular etching, high definition, VASER

Enhancing the abdominal wall due to aging and weight changes are one of the most common concerns on the daily practice of the aesthetic surgeon. Achieving a muscular, toned, and athletic-looking body is synonymous with health, youth, and beauty. Now it is becoming the goal of body contouring as well.

21.1 Female versus Male Anatomy: Landmarks, Planes, and Superficial Anatomy

The abdominal contour identity is given mainly by the appearance of the "rectus abdominis" muscle. It is a vertically oriented pair of strap muscles that run along the central part of the anterior abdominal wall arising from the pubic symphysis, crest, and pecten of the pubis and goes upwards to insert into the xiphoid process and costal cartilages of the fifth to seventh ribs. Inferiorly is covered only on its anterior surface by the rectus sheath, and above the arcuate line is covered on both sides by the rectus sheath.

The surface anatomy can be easily palpated in slim patients. The muscular intersections divide the muscle into segments that create individual muscular bellies otherwise commonly referred to as the six-pack.

The Thoracic arch forms an angle of about 90 degrees in males and 60 degrees in females being more rounded in males due to the highest tendinous intersection of rectus abdominis medially.

The umbilicus lies within a defect in the linea alba at the level of the fourth lumbar vertebra. In athletic males, a sharp rim is usually present at the upper border of the umbilicus, whereas the lower border is less well defined. In females, a peri-umbilical fat pad deepens the navel and obscures its borders.

There is a clear structural and functional division of the fat layers: A superficial, dense-packed with a vertical and organized structure metabolically stable less prompt to changes with the weight variations; A deep fat layer separated by the Scarpa's fascia, containing a less organized fat tissue where most of the fat is deposited.

21.2 Steady versus Fluctuating Beauty Standards

The female ideal biotype is not a static concept; it constantly changes influenced by fashion, cultural trends, age, ethnicity, and other tendencies. In the last half-century it has had dramatic changes.

After World War II with the return to a healthier lifestyle, the curvy, hourglass shape with more importance given to the breast size and little attention to the waist was the ideal.

During the 60s everything changed, with the empowerment of the women's liberation movements, women start to take part in the social and political life, the miniskirt was the official trend and the curvy woman was not the ideal anymore, the popular Twiggy model leads to a thinner body image with long legs, chic bodies, and outfits.

The 70s were a reaction against the established patterns in social, political, and of course aesthetics could not escape from this. Hippie trends took place; the informal look was the rule.

The 80s were the birth of the supermodel era: a sexy, curvy, and pretty woman could be rich, famous, and successful just because of the way she looked. Women everywhere found this as the ideal and started to look forward to imitating them.

The 90s woman was known as the "junkie" chick. The new idea was the "thinner the better," up to a point that the health started to be a serious concern and an anorexia epidemic started to grow.

The big question to ask nowadays is what the woman wants. The answer can only be addressed based on distinctive aspects: the geographic location, age, fashion trends, and ethnicity. Younger women tend to search for an athletic body type while one after giving birth tends to look for a more subtle look. Asian women prefer to have a rounded face (full moon) while occidental women like a defined, bony, square-like face.

For males, the ideal body biotype has been almost the same throughout time. Artwork from different 'cultures and times share the same concept about the ideal male body, from ancient Greek and Roman, the Renaissance masters, and even the contemporary movements. The ideal of athletic must have a very well-defined muscle figure that implies youth, vitality, and health.

21.3 Biotypes and the Influence Results

Sheldon in the 1940s defined three body somatotypes to classify the body and fat tendency.

21.3.1 Ectomorphs

These individuals have scant body fat and muscle, they are usually tall, flat chested, lack curves, and not easy to gain weight. Psychologists also give them some personality trends towards anxiety.

21.3.2 Endomorphs

They easily store higher amounts of fat tissue, muscle, and gain weight easily.

21.3.3 Mesomorphs

They are athletic, strong with an adequate amount of fat, and easily gain or lose weight without too much effort.

Knowing the somatotype or body biotype is the main factor for choosing the type of abdominal high definition, but always having as target outcome the athletic mesomorph body type. In the overweight patient, the main focus of the surgery is to remove as much fat as possible. If the patient is already slim or athletic, the fat removal will be slight and the purpose to reshape, not to "de-bulk". For those patients, we will also transfer fat to the muscles to increase their definition.

21.4 Male High Definition in the Abdominal Area: Procedure, Variations According to Bio Types

21.4.1 The Markings

The correct abdominal marking is an essential part of the technique. Markings are done in three layers. All markings should be done with the patient in standing position. The use of markers with different colors is advisable.

The marks for deep layer liposuction are done in the areas where extra fat is commonly located especially in the infra-umbilical zone.

For the framing look for the costal margin, the supra-umbilical, the linea alba, the lateral borders of the rectus abdominis muscles, and if possible, the transverse inscriptions of it, in thin and athletic patients, should not be a problem.

In the obese patient custom markings and different positioning are necessary to accurately make the marking. In these patients there are two main scenarios: (1) Predominance of intra-abdominal fat content, and (2) Predominance of the extra-abdominal fat content.

The main fat extraction in male obese patients will vary also according to the presence of intra vs. extra abdominal fat. In patients with extra-abdominal fat, the resection is focused on the lower abdomen and retraction is highly encouraged by performing a lot of superficial fat resection.

In patients with intra-abdominal fat, the resection is performed in the extra-abdominal fat but procuring to remove the central area to diminish the curvature of the anterior abdomen. As the intra-abdominal fat cannot be reached by liposuction, a strict diet low-carb after the surgery should be followed to reduce this fat.

21.5 The Negative Spaces

The negative spaces are areas that form the shadows of the superficial anatomy. As we have already marked the areas of superficial and deep liposuction, connecting these two layers would make this an intermediate layer of markings. There are specific areas of negative spaces:
• The area below the oblique and transverse muscles.
• The area following the midline supra-umbilical marking.

- The areas between the transverse inscriptions of the rectus muscle.
- The areas between the superolateral border of the rectus abdominis muscle and the lower border of the pectoralis muscle.
- The area between the lateral border of the pectoralis m. and the lateral latissimus dorsi m.

21.5.1 Incisions

The position of the incisions is critical to easily and safely reach the entire area but at the same time be hidden and provide the patient no stigmata of the surgery whenever the patient shows the body. We recommend the following access ports:
- Below the pubic hairline, two incisions in the same line of the vertical semilunaris lines to provide access to most of the abdominal area, including the flank area and waistline, also the rectus abdominis sheets.
- Umbilical incision to provide access to the inferior abdominal area, vertical midline above the umbilicus and the central and supra-umbilical area.
- Inferior nipple incision in men provides good access to the pectoralis area, the superior abdomen and the superior flank area and the axilla.
- Inframammary crease incision following the lateral border of the rectus abdominis muscle over the fold mark. This incision provides access to the superior abdomen and flanks. In women, if the breast is not big enough to create the fold, we should avoid this incision as much as possible because the scar may be too visible, an areolar scar could be a good option instead.
- Additional incisions must be needed when the fatty tissue is excessive, they could be performed on anterior axillary fold and the midline in the pubis. Incisions over the abdominal area must be avoided, but if needed, they could be done over the horizontal marks of the abdominis muscle.

21.5.2 Infiltration

The infiltration is done using a solution of 1000 mL Ringer's lactate, 1:100.000 epinephrine and lidocaine 20 mL 1% solution following a 2:1 ratio, first in the deep and later in the superficial layer.

21.5.3 Emulsification

Beginning in the superficial layer, the VASER probe must be applied with a smooth movement, tuned into pulsed mode to prevent heat generation. Additional VASER time would be required for the framing areas. Then proceed on the deep layer. Begin with the deepest areas to ensure full emulsification, rubbing the probe against the muscular layer. This will ensure to extract all the fat in this layer. Go progressively making your way up to reach again the superficial layer.

21.5.4 Extraction

It must begin in the deep abdominal area focusing on the infra-umbilical zone trying to empty the whole anterior abdomen until leaving a 1 cm thickness flap. Then continue with the deep area of the flanks until reach a 0.5 cm thickness flap.

21.6 The Rectus Abdominis

Start with the horizontal inscriptions. Unless requested to achieve a fit appearance, avoid this on the female patient. Work on the horizontal inscriptions with: (1) Directly or parallel to the incision point, which means that there will be incision per each section of the six-pack, at least three; (2) Directly using curved cannulas, with the right tools would be efficient enough saving some incisions, and (3) Indirectly, performing the inscription perpendicular to the incision point. Using small (3 mm), this maneuver can be used for creating the line or as adjunctive to the other two maneuvers.

Start with a small cannula (3.0 mm), either straight or curved. Usually the umbilical incision one is the one to begin. Start very superficial, and later make your way deep, until the groove is formed. Proceed to the upper ones, mostly they can be done through the nipple incisions, if not, an incision can be one over the line of the lower 2nd horizontal inscription. Always do the same inscription from several access points; the ideal is to criss-cross the inscriptions from three points.

Leave the midline for last, taking care of not to overdo it when doing the horizontal inscriptions. Make sure that you finished the work over the inscriptions before moving into the midline. Use a 3.0 mm cannula and move later to a 3.7 mm for deepening the midline.

21.7 The Intermediate Layer Liposuction

This step of the surgery is critical to achieve an optimal high definition lipoplasty. The artistry of making a carved fat into a shape that looks and feels natural takes its origins in how the light is going to affect the shapes. By turning lines into curves and making shadows along the natural ones in the anatomy, the results will be better than expected.

Begin by doing the negative space in the subcostal space keeping in mind that this area always moves from the standing position to the decubitus, so keep the one you marked in standing. Then proceed to the space below the pectoralis, always from different access points: the nipple incision contralateral and the axillary incision. Last, do the triangle between the pectoralis and the anterior border of the lattisimus dorsi.

21.8 Adjunctive Fat Grafting in the Torso: Where and When To Use It

The use of fat grafting is reserved for what we call alpha muscles. These are the group of muscles that give the appearance of power, meaning that they need to be bigger to enhance the athletic look. In the upper torso the main muscle considered an alpha is the pectoralis muscle. The rectus abdominis muscle is more important in the sense of definition rather than volume. So, regarding the rectus abdominis muscle by doing fat grafting only will make it look awkward. There are very few indications for fat grafting in this area. The first one is when in a secondary patient we see an over resection—due to a previous liposuction—over the central portion of the abdomen, the second is when we perform a full lipoabdominoplasty and high-definition in a male patient: we need to re-create the six-pack without compromising the vascularization of the flap.

21.9 Complications, Prevention, and Treatment

Seroma is the more frequently reported complication. It is improved with adequate postsurgical care and the use of drains in the in the inguinal area in male patients, and in the sacral in females. Nearly all seromas can be managed with serial percutaneous drainage without the need of surgical treatment.

Surgical site Infections at entrance ports occur rarely and usually have an excellent response to oral antibiotics and local wound care.

The incidence of contour irregularities and skin burns due to VASER are associate with the surgeon-learning curve; many irregularities require a secondary procedure to be corrected. The burns can be avoided with the adequate infiltration in the port site, skin protection with ports and surgical towels as well as an adequate VASER time.

The skin induration can be avoided by the adequate usage of the VASER probe by the use of low power pulse mode (60%).

Suggested Readings

Hoyos AE, Prendergast PM. High definition body sculpting. Springer; 2014

Hoyos AE, Millard JA. VASER-assisted high-definition liposculpture. Aesthet Surg J 2007;27(6):594–604

Sheldon, William H. The varieties of human pshysique: an introduction to constitutional psychology. Harper & Brothers; 1940

22 Flanks and Hips

Spero J. Theodorou

Abstract

The flanks and hips are the most commonly treated areas for liposuction. This is likely due to the forgiving nature of this anatomic subunit and the high level of patient satisfaction. To that end, these areas are commonly treated alone or in conjunction with other body contouring procedures like abdominoplasty. To achieve optimal aesthetic results, the surgeon must understand the anatomic differences between men and women in this region of the body. The surgeon must also be aware of potential asymmetries that a patient may present with preoperatively. In this chapter, we offer our technique for successfully and efficiently treating the flanks and hips in both men and women. In addition, we review our postoperative protocol and strategies for managing postoperative complications.

Keywords: Body contouring, liposuction, hips, flanks, love handles, VASER, radiofrequency, RF, radiofrequency-assisted liposuction, RFAL

22.1 Introduction

Flanks and hips are the most commonly treated areas for liposuction in men and women. They also have the distinction of being one of the areas with the highest satisfaction level when treated with liposuction. Treatment of these areas was popularized in the late 1970s by Teimourian and Fisher and the term "flank curettage" was coined.[1] By the 1990s, Pitman reported that 45% of his patients had these areas treated with virtually all abdominoplasties as standard adjunctive therapy.[2] The common term used now days are "love handles."

22.2 Anatomy

The fat in these areas is divided into superficial and deep. The superficial fascial system (SFS) is responsible for encasing the superficial fat.[3] It consists of an intertwined fibro-septal network (FSN) consisting of fascial elements that provide structural support to the fat as well as to the overlying dermis. The superficial fat tends to be more structured in nature due to this fascial network, whereas the deeper fat contains less fascial elements.

The FSN's role as a support pillar for the overlying dermis comes into play in cases requiring dermal tightening utilizing radiofrequency-assisted liposuction.[4] Elements of the Superficial Fascial System (SFS) condense down to the level of the muscle fascia and form Lockwood's zones of adherence. This deep fat compartment is defined in men as cephalad to the iliac crest and has implications in the treatment of the flanks. In women, it tends to overly the iliac crest and hence lies more inferior (▶Fig. 22.1).

Lastly, the anatomical implication for treatment that needs to be taken into consideration is the underlying skeletal framework. Clinical conditions such as scoliosis, and the degree of pelvic tilt can have impact on the physical appearance of the fat distribution in the flanks. Patients will often mention their "bigger side" vs. "smaller side." Therefore, it is of paramount importance that these asymmetries be pointed out to the patient on the preoperative photographs prior to surgery. What patients and physicians often surmise as a

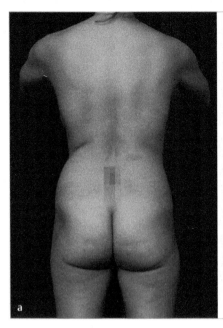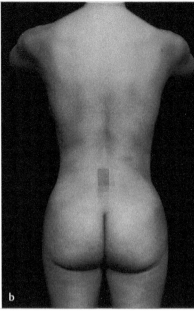

Fig. 22.1 (a, b) A 38-year-old female who underwent bilateral flank liposuction utilizing Vaser at 60% power Vaser mode with autologous fat grafting of each buttock of 350 cc. Procedure was performed under local anesthesia. Brazilian Butt-lift Under Local Anesthesia (BBULA).

bigger vs. smaller side can simply be a manifestation of the underlying skeletal framework and not a quantitative judgment on fat amount. It's important to explain to the patient in the preoperative consultation that while every effort will be made to attempt the correction of such asymmetry, it is typically not guaranteed (▶Fig. 22.1).

22.3 Markings

The patient is examined in the upright position and the arms are held out at full extension (▶Fig. 22.2a, b). The iliac crest is palpated, identified, and marked. A single access point is marked cephalad to this point and should be well hidden within a bathing suit or underwear. The superior border is then marked at the 8–10th rib. The patient is rotated clockwise and the posterior border of the resection is identified approximately 5–10 cm from the midline. A vertical line is dropped from this point to 5–10 cm above the buttock crease. This point is connected and intersects the lateral single access incision and forms the inferior border of the resection. The marking continues anteriorly and tapers off at the level of the anterior axillary line. The superior border of the resection ends at the anterior axillary line. This determines the extent of the flank resection (▶Fig. 22.4a, b).

22.4 Positioning

Since the flank extends posteriorly from the back all the way to the anterior axillary line the optimal position for treatment is the lateral decubitus position (▶Fig. 22.2). This allows for full visualization of the flank as opposed to the supine or prone position. One of the advantages of local anesthesia is that the patient can assist with positioning. If the patient is undergoing general anesthesia a gel-based prop is used to keep the patient in this position. Only a circulating assistant is required in both cases.

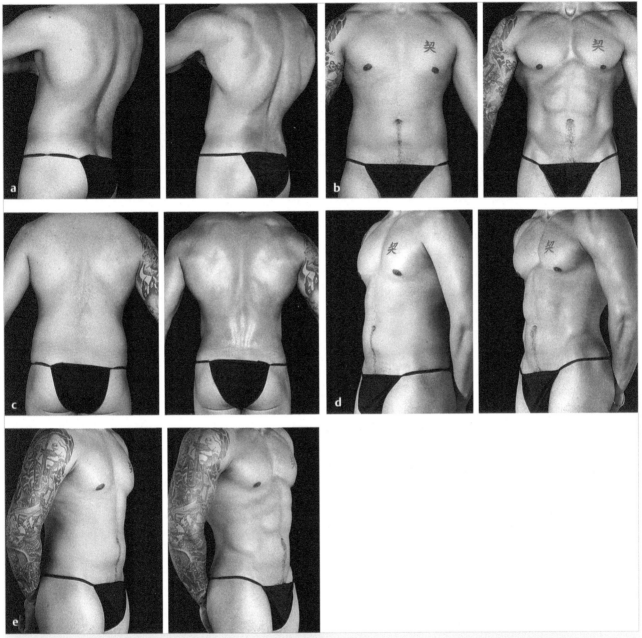

Fig. 22.2 (a–e) A 30-year-old male having undergone high definition body sculpting with Vaser of the abdomen and flanks.

22.5 Treatment

All treatment is performed through a single access incision. Care must be taken not to over resect the area of entry. In males, ultrasound-assisted liposuction, VASER is used as the fat is more fibrous and tends to be bloodier in nature. The combination of 1.5 mg Epinephrine in the tumescent and the emulsification aspects of the ultrasound energy typically alleviate the above issues. A single ring Vaser probe is inserted through a single access incision after the protective port is secured into place. The protective ports are critical as they protect the skin from the heat generated from the probe and would otherwise result in a burn to the skin. The energy is set on Vaser mode between 70–100% power depending on the size of the area to be treated and the thickness of the flap. Typical treatment time ranges from 5–7 minutes. Male patients tend to respond very well to these treatment settings as it not only allows for a more aggressive approach in regards to fat resection but has the added benefit of less postoperative bruising and swelling (▶ Fig. 22.3).

For females, we tend to use a gentler three-ring probe set at 70% Vaser mode since the fat tends to be more areolar and not as fibrous. The endpoint is felt as loss of resistance of the ultrasound probe gliding through the tissues. Once this is achieved it is safe to assume that emulsification is complete. Most surgeons typically allow a timeline of 7–13 minutes (if not longer) for the epinephrine in the tumescent to have an effect. This time block can be used for application of the ultrasound energy. The argument presented by some that ultrasound energy treatment takes more operative time thus goes away. Radiofrequency-assisted liposuction (Bodytite) is only used in this area should the operator wish to obtain added tightening. Since this is an area of adherence the skin tends to contract quite well with traditional methods of liposuction. Most importantly, we have found that the combination of Vaser energy, Epinephrine 1.5 mg in the tumescent solution and slow deliberate infiltration performed under local anesthesia can contribute to faster recovery times with less bruising and swelling (▶ Fig. 22.4).

The endpoint for use of the Vaser is loss of resistance and is gauged as an effortless gliding of the probe through the tissues. Once the endpoint is achieved, a 4–0 mm double Mercedes PAL cannula is used for debulking of the deep fat compartment followed by a 3–0 mm double Mercedes PAL cannula for superficial fat resection. The final stage is typically performed with a 3–0 mm Wells Johnson double Mercedes manual cannula for superficial subdermal liposuction. This is often reserved for male and Fitzpatrick III–V skin types as the fat tends to be more adherent to the dermis in these patients. Treatment of this area with PAL alone can result in a substandard underwhelming result. The endpoint for contouring is an even thickness flap with no irregularities. The access point is closed with a 5–0 Nylon and removed at 10 days postoperatively.

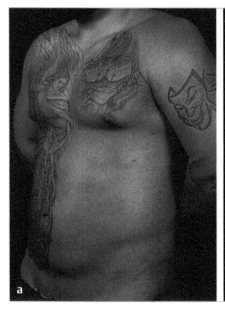 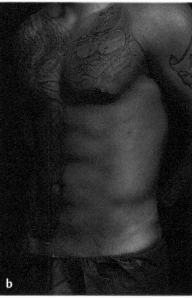

Fig. 22.3 (a, b) A 28-year-old male having undergone high definition body sculpting of the abdomen and flanks. The flank area is seen blending into the lateral abdomen making the lateral decubitus position during surgery very important for proper evaluation and treatment.

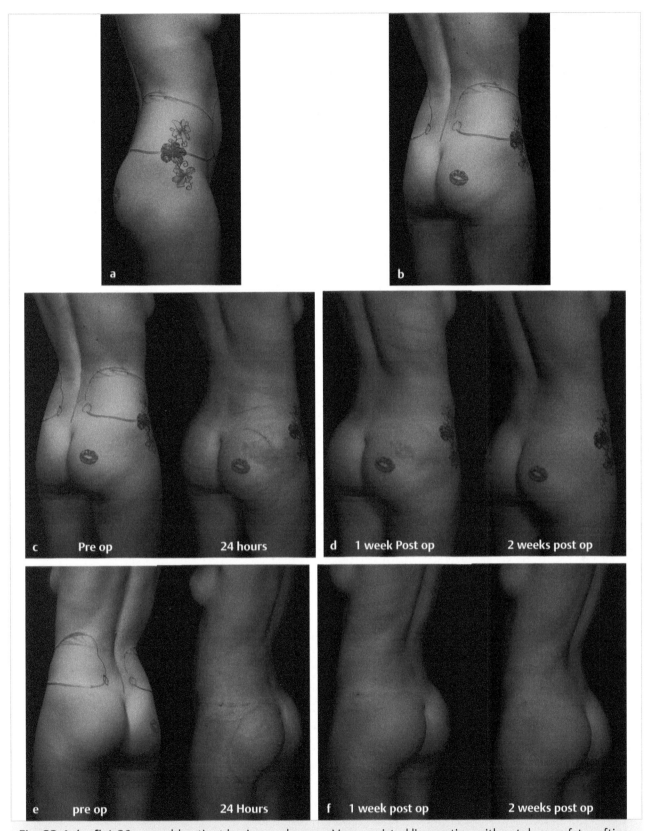

Fig. 22.4 (a–f) A 28-year-old patient having undergone Vaser assisted liposuction with autologous fat grafting of 500 cc to each buttock under local anesthesia. The timing of the postoperative course is noted as well as the evidence of minimal bruising and swelling.

22.6 Postoperative Care

Garment compression is used for two weeks followed by Spanx (SPANX Inc. Atlanta, Georgia) for another 4 weeks should the patient desire faster resolution of the postoperative edema. Numbness is an often expected sequella in this area and can last up to six months. The patient should be informed of this possibility prior to the procedure.

22.7 Complications

The flanks as a general rule are a forgiving area. Removal of fat from the deep compartment alone will guarantee an aesthetically pleasing result. Patients with Fitzpatrick Skin III and higher that exhibit thicker dermis warrant a more aggressive approach with judicious removal of fat from the superficial compartment. Care must be taken to avoid contour deformities when performing this type of subdermal liposuction. The most common contour deformity after flank suction tends to be remaining fat left behind over the 8th–10th rib. Patients will complain that instead of a smooth transition from the back to the waist there is bulge overlying their rib cage. In order to alleviate this problem, care must be taken during the procedure to go up and above this rib to remove the fat for proper feathering purposes.

Energy-related complications from VASER such as periportal burns should be treated conservatively with local wound care. In the event of second degree burns with radiofrequency-assisted liposuction, excision, and closure are recommended for an optimal healing result as these tend to be full thickness in nature.

References

[1] Teimourian B, Fisher JB. Suction curettage to remove excess fat for body contouring. Plast Reconstr Surg 1981;68(1):50–58
[2] Pitman G. Liposuction and aesthetic surgery. St. Louis: QMP; Copyright 1993
[3] Lockwood TE. Superficial fascial system (SFS) of the trunk and extremities: a new concept. Plast Reconstr Surg 1991;87(6):1009–1018
[4] Theodorou SJ, Paresi R, Chia CT. Radiofrequency-assisted liposuction device for body contouring: 97 patients under local anesthesia. Aesthetic Plastic Surgery

23 Gluteal Augmentation with Implants

Douglas Senderoff

Abstract

This chapter discusses the use of solid silicone implants in buttock augmentation including patient evaluation, preoperative planning, surgical technique, management of common complications and revisional buttock implant surgery. Intramuscular and subfascial implant placement along with the advantages and disadvantages of both techniques are discussed. Recommendations for achieving successful outcomes are presented along with relevant citations from the scientific literature. Case examples with photographs are included illustrating the results of gluteal augmentation with implants.

Keywords: Buttock implants, gluteal implants, buttock augmentation, gluteal augmentation, buttock enhancement, revision buttock augmentation, buttock implant complication

---

Key Points

- Biodimensional planning is essential to obtaining good results.
- Select an implant that will produce the maximum point of projection at the correct level.
- Avoid implants greater than 350 cc in primary implant surgery.
- Choose the insertion plane best suited for the patient.
- Ensure that the wound closure is tension-free.
- Recognize and act on complications as soon as possible.
- Be prepared to remove implants early in case of infection.
- Patient compliance with limited activity in the postoperative period is essential.
- Implant replacement after infection can be performed after 6 months.

23.1 Patient Evaluation

The evaluation of a potential candidate for gluteal augmentation begins with an assessment of several anatomic variables which determine the suitability for surgery and affect the potential results. The underlying shape of the pelvis and spine although not part of the augmentation procedure should be considered. The pelvis may present limitations on the size of the implant as a narrow pelvis will require an implant of less base diameter than would fit in a wide pelvis. The spine should be examined to look for preexisting asymmetries that may affect the results. The shape and volume of the buttocks are mostly determined by the gluteal musculature along with the amount and distribution of subcutaneous fat. Understanding the contribution of the muscle and fat specific to each patient is an important part of evaluating potential candidates for gluteal augmentation.[1] The skin of the buttock region should be evaluated in terms of thickness, elasticity, and position relative to the infragluteal fold. Patients with skin laxity and infragluteal fold ptosis may require a buttock lift or direct fold excision in order to obtain an acceptable result. An understanding of the anatomy of the gluteal region is essential in the evaluation and planning of surgery (▶ Fig. 23.1).[2,3,4]

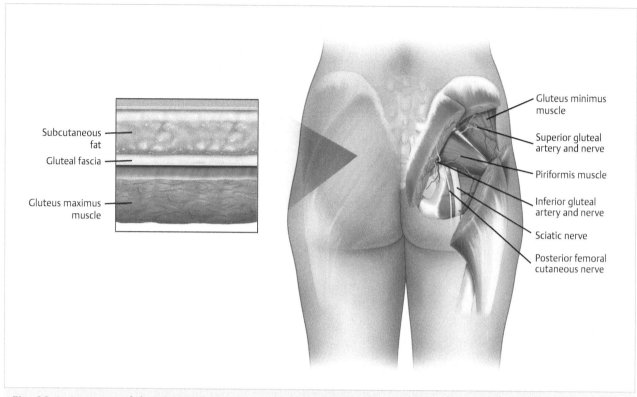

Fig. 23.1 Anatomy of the gluteus maximus muscle and deeper structure.

The practical approach to evaluating a patient presenting for buttock augmentation using an implant involves choosing the type of implant and the plane of insertion. The choice of implant between round and oval and the plane of insertion of either subfascial or intramuscular depends on three anatomic variables. The first anatomic variable requiring attention is the length of the buttock. A patient with a long buttock would be more suitable with an oval anatomic implant. A round implant placed in a long buttock would likely leave the bottom third of the buttock empty. A short buttock would be more suited towards a round implant since an implant with an appropriately sized base diameter would fill all areas of the buttock. Implant position can be determined through evaluation of the second anatomic variable which is the amount and quality of subcutaneous fat. A patient with thick subcutaneous fat would likely have enough soft tissue to conceal a subfascial buttock implant. Patients with minimal buttock subcutaneous fat would benefit from intramuscular implant placement to avoid complications such as palpability and visibility. In patients with inadequate soft tissue of the buttock gluteal implant placement is not advisable. The third anatomic variable of skin laxity should be evaluated to determine the need for skin excision. Moderate buttock skin laxity is likely to require infragluteal fold excision after buttock implant surgery while severe buttock skin laxity should be managed with a buttock lift prior to implant placement.

It is important for surgeons who perform buttock augmentation to be familiar with both techniques of intramuscular and subfascial implant placement.[5,6] The history of buttock augmentation with implants dates back to 1969 with the insertion of a round breast implant through an infragluteal fold incision to correct left gluteal muscle atrophy.[7] Cosmetic gluteoplasty was first described in 1973 by placing implants in the subcutaneous plane.[8] The choice of incision including bilateral supragluteal, infragluteal fold, and the intergluteal crease was described in 1977.[9,10] The intramuscular implant is more difficult to insert as the dissection plane is indistinct and often bloody. In addition, intramuscular placement can result in lack of inferior fullness if the inferior pole is not dissected enough. Intramuscular implant placement has been shown to result in as much as a 6.4% atrophy of the gluteus maximus muscle with a subsequent return of strength.[11] The advantage of intramuscular placement is less palpability, less visibility, and less infragluteal fold stretching. The complication rates after intramuscular placement were found to be lower than other pocket locations.[12] The subfascial technique is based on the ability of the gluteal aponeurosis to hold the implants in position.[13] The subfascial technique has the advantage of an easier and distinct dissection plane with less blood loss along with a more global buttock enhancement with greater projection.[14] The disadvantage of subfascial placement in thin patients is implant palpability and visibility of the edges and possible infragluteal fold displacement.

After examining a patient presenting for consultation for gluteal implants the surgeon must decide whether the patient is a good candidate for surgery. The ideal candidate for gluteal implants is a normoweight patient in good health with sufficient buttock soft tissue to support and conceal an implant. Indications for buttock augmentation with an implant include: lack of volume, poor projection, asymmetry, contour deformity, and limited availability of fat for transfer (▶ Fig. 23.2). Contraindications to buttock implant surgery include: inadequate soft tissue, general or local infection, unrealistic expectations, psychological instability, and diabetics on insulin. Precautions to buttock implant surgery include: autoimmune disease, poor wound healing, BMI greater than 30, prior buttock injections, and a history of radiation to the buttocks.[15]

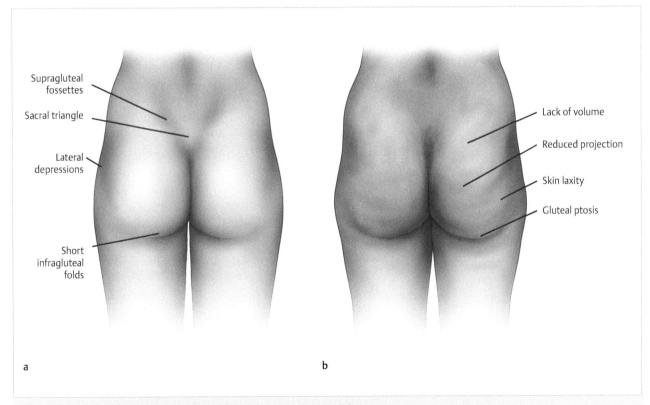

Fig. 23.2 **(a)** Ideal surface anatomy **(b)** Gluteoplasty candidate

23.2 Preoperative Planning and Preparation

When planning buttock implant surgery it is important to first define patient expectations in order to determine whether these expectations can be met. After an evaluation of the anatomic variables of the buttock and determining implant shape and placement and potential need for skin lift the potential choice of implants can be presented to the patient. Having sample implants of varying shapes and sizes is essential to precise preoperative planning. Biodimensional analysis with consideration of the buttock base diameter and length and capacity for volume expansion should be exercised when choosing the appropriate buttock implant. The limitations of implant size should be communicated to the patient during the planning stage of surgery. It is important to only use an implant that is appropriately sized to the dimensions of the patient. Attempting to insert an implant that is overly large in order to satisfy patient desires is counterproductive and can result in complications. Implants over 350 cc should not be inserted by the inexperienced buttock implant surgeon. During the preoperative examination, the implant sizer is placed over the buttock at the desired point of maximal projection to determine suitability. By placing the sizer on the patient, a determination can be made whether to use an oval or round implant by the amount of lower buttock that is covered by the implant sizer. If the lower pole is not adequately addressed with a round implant an oval anatomic implant should be considered. For patients who desire large volume augmentations the risk of wound healing complications should be emphasized. These patients would benefit from insertion of an appropriately sized implant and offered an implant exchange to a larger size after a minimum of 6 months when the capsule is formed and stable.

The patient can prepare for surgery by cleansing the surgical site with Chlorhexidine the night before and the morning of surgery. A light low residue diet is recommended prior to surgery. A bowel prep is not necessary. Preoperative labs and medical clearance are obtained for those patients with medical concerns.

23.3 Surgical Technique

The patient is marked in the upright position by placing the appropriate implant sizer over the desired maximum point of projection of the buttock which usually corresponds to the level of the pubis. The sizer is then outlined with a surgical marker. Areas of liposuction or fat grafting are marked if necessary. The patient is placed on a stretcher and undergoes either general endotracheal, epidural, or spinal anesthesia. Bolsters and placed under the hips and chest and the patient is positioned prone on the operating table. A urinary catheter is inserted if the expected length of surgery is over 3 hours. Sequential compression devices are placed on the lower extremities. A surgical scrub of the buttocks is done followed by a surgical prep with either povidone iodine or chlorhexidine and alcohol. A rolled-up laparotomy sponge is placed over the anus followed by draping. The use of a barrier drape such as Ioban (3M, St. Paul, MN) is recommended to reduce potential intraoperative wound contamination. A dose of Cefazolin is administered intravenously prior to skin incision. The markings are infiltrated with 1% lidocaine with epinephrine. A single 6.5 cm midline intergluteal incision is made down to the sacral fascia ending inferiorly at the level of the coccyx. Surveys of American and international surgeons revealed a preference for the single midline incision.[16,17] Another acceptable incision is the bilateral parasacral incision which leaves an intact area of midline intergluteal skin for closure. After making the intergluteal incision dissection is performed laterally exposing the gluteus maximus fascia. The fascia is then incised parallel to the intergluteal skin incision exposing the gluteus maximus (▶Fig. 23.3). Subfascial undermining is then performed with the aid of a lighted fiberoptic retractor and long tip electrocautery. The use of a specially designed gluteal retractor can aid in the dissection by placing downward pressure on the gluteal musculature thereby creating a better optical cavity (▶Fig. 23.4). The dissection is continued until the limits of the external skin markings are reached. Perforating blood vessels can be coagulated with the use of an insulated forceps. The subfascial dissection should be precise and mostly bloodless. It is important to not over dissect laterally or inferiorly to avoid potential migration and malposition of the implant. After dissection is complete the wound is rinsed with an antimicrobial solution of either povidone iodine and saline or antibiotics. Hemostasis is obtained and the wound is re-prepped. The implant is rinsed in antibiotic solution and then placed into the subfascial space through the intergluteal wound. It is important to position the implants far enough away from the midline so that a tension-free closure can be performed. Closed suction drains are not usually necessary. Wound closure is then begun by tacking each side of the incision to the midline sacral fascia and periosteum. Layered wound closure is then continued with absorbable sutures and a running intracuticular suture.

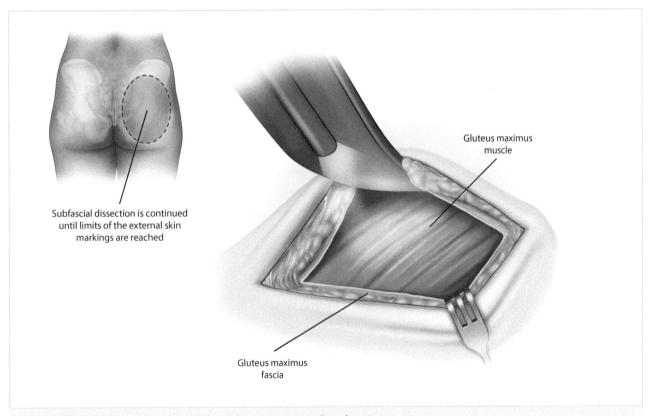

Subfascial dissection is continued until limits of the external skin markings are reached

Gluteus maximus muscle

Gluteus maximus fascia

Fig. 23.3 Initial dissection for subfascial or intramuscular placement.

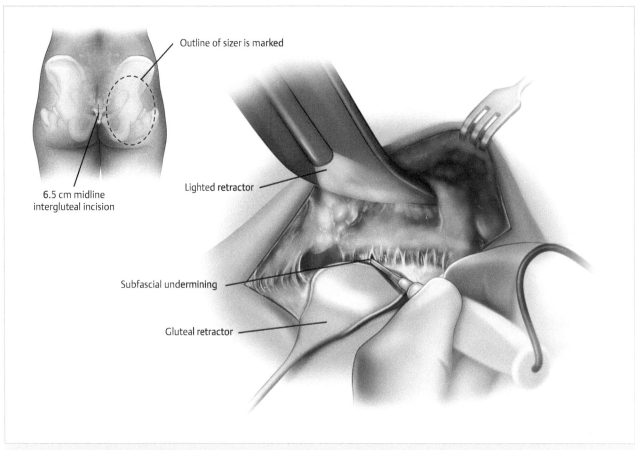

Outline of sizer is marked

6.5 cm midline
intergluteal incision

Lighted retractor

Subfascial undermining

Gluteal retractor

Fig. 23.4 Subfascial gluteal dissection.

The intramuscular technique begins with subfascial dissection exposing the gluteus maximus for 7 cm on both sides of the midline incision. The gluteus maximus is then divided parallel to the direction of its muscle fibers to a depth of 2–3 cm. A mostly blunt dissection plane is then established using a blunt dissector and a fiberoptic retractor. A long smooth tip insulated forceps is used to coagulate perforating intramuscular blood vessels. The inferior portion and the superior portion of the intramuscular pocket should be at the same depth and result in the creation of one continuous intramuscular space 2–3 cm thick of sufficient size to accommodate the desired implant.[18,19] It is important not to over dissect laterally to avoid implant displacement. Care must be taken to avoid perforating the gluteus maximus muscle when dissecting laterally as the muscle curves downward toward the hip.[20] After completion of the dissection laparotomy pads are placed into the newly created intramuscular space to check the adequacy of dissection and to check hemostasis. Laparotomy pads are then removed and adjustments to the dissection can be made. The wound is then rinsed with antibiotic solution. The wound is re-prepped and the implants are placed into the intramuscular space and positioned appropriately. Drains are often used as the blunt muscle dissection results in bleeding. The gluteus maximus is closed securely over the implant with either a continuous running absorbable or permanent suture. The midline incision is then closed in layers as described earlier (▶ Fig. 23.5).

After the completion of surgery the patient is placed on a stretcher and awakened from anesthesia. Compression shorts are applied. The patient is

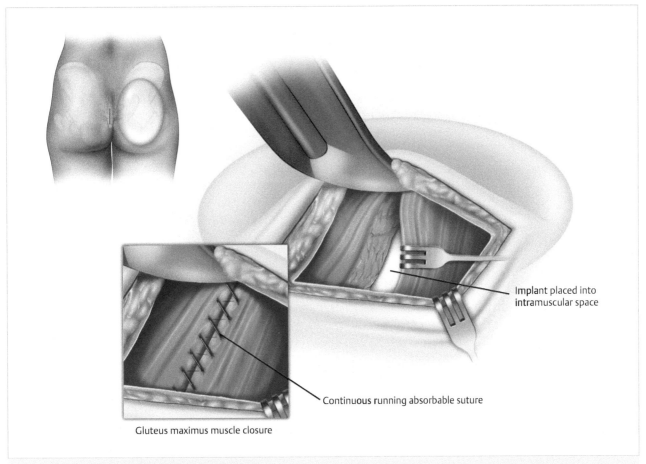

Implant placed into
intramuscular space

Continuous running absorbable suture

Gluteus maximus muscle closure

Fig. 23.5 Intramuscular implant placement.

then brought to the recovery area and placed in the prone position until discharge.

Patients are advised to recover at home in the prone position as much as possible for the first week. Sitting should be avoided for 2–3 weeks if possible. Compression shorts are recommended for 3 weeks. Early ambulation is recommended to avoid deep vein thrombosis but strenuous activity is discouraged. Exercise can be resumed in 6–8 weeks. Muscle relaxants may prove beneficial in patients undergoing intramuscular implant placement. Oral antibiotics are used according to surgeon preference. Drains are removed when less than 25 mL of fluid is obtained in a 24-hour period. If the drainage does not subside or fluid accumulates after drain removal a sample of periprosthetic fluid should be sent for culture. If infection is suspected antibiotic therapy can be initiated and then adjusted after the results of the culture are obtained.

Ancillary surgical procedures that can enhance the results of buttock augmentation include liposuction, fat grafting, buttock lift, and excision of the infragluteal fold. Liposuction of the lower back can improve the waist to hip (WHR) ratio to produce a more desirable proportion.[21,22,23] A WHR quotient of 0.7 in women is widely accepted as a standard of beauty.[24] In men, liposuction of the lower back and flanks can create a more attractive result. Fat grafting can add additional volume to the buttocks and create a smooth transition between the buttock implant and the lateral thighs and hips. Liposuction with fat grafting can be safely performed at the time of buttock implantation or later on to add volume or correct contour irregularities.[25] In patients with severe laxity of the buttocks infragluteal fold excision or buttock lift may be performed prior to implantation. In patients with mild buttock skin laxity a reassessment of the buttock skin 3 months after implantation is advisable. At this time, precise correction of the infragluteal fold may be safely performed. Markings for infragluteal fold excision are performed in the upright position taking care to place the scar in the new infragluteal fold. After full-thickness skin excision the wound is closed in multiple layers without wide undermining of the wound edges. It is important to tack the wound margins to the fascia to secure the position of the new infragluteal crease. The goal of the skin excision is to create a buttock that is rounder, tighter, and more youthful appearing. Drains are not required. Compression shorts are applied and patients are instructed to recover in the prone position. Sitting is to be avoided for 2–3 weeks.

23.4 Complications

It is important for surgeons who perform buttock augmentation with implants to be able to recognize and manage the common complications of this surgery. Most of the complications of buttock augmentation occur in the early postoperative period and should be diagnosed and managed promptly in order to avoid additional problems.

Infection requiring implant removal can occur within the first week of surgery as evidenced by erythema, swelling, pain, and fluctuance of the buttock. Antibiotic therapy should be initiated if infection is suspected. Needle aspiration of the buttock with fluid culture is essential in confirming the diagnosis of implant infection. While early cellulitis may be managed with antibiotic therapy it is unlikely that an implant may be salvaged once a fluid culture from the periprosthetic space shows evidence of bacterial growth. In this circumstance, the implant should be removed and the wound should be irrigated with antibiotic solution and a drain inserted. If the infection is confined to the periprosthetic space the intergluteal wound may be closed after implant removal. Bilateral implant removal is not necessary if the infection is unilateral. Staphylococcus aureus was the most commonly isolated pathogen in the author's series of buttock implant infections. Published reports of implant infection rates vary from 1 to 7%.[17,26,27]

Wound dehiscence which has been reported between 6 and 30% is a largely avoidable complication of buttock augmentation with implants.[26,28,29] Implant selection is one cause of wound dehiscence. It is not recommended to use an implant greater than 350 cc in primary implant surgery by inexperienced surgeons in order to minimize this complication. There were no instances of wound dehiscence in a published series using implants between 250–350 cc.[30] Tension-free wound closure through using appropriately sized implants and securely tacking each side of the intergluteal wound to the sacral fascia is essential to ensuring successful wound healing.

Hematoma can occur early in the postoperative period and can be managed in several ways. A buttock that is firm, fluctuant, painful and discolored requires operative exploration. The implant should be removed and placed in antibiotic solution and the wound should be evacuated of all blood and then irrigated. Sources of bleeding should be controlled although an obvious source of bleeding may not be identifiable. The implant can be replaced and a drain should be utilized. A small hematoma as evidenced by slight fluctuance and minor discomfort can be managed with serial aspiration until resolved. The semi-solid nature of the implant allows for needle aspiration without risk of implant damage. Large hematomas should be addressed promptly to avoid further complications such as wound dehiscence, infection, and asymmetry.

Seroma formation most often occurs early in the postoperative period and may present as a warm, fluctuant, asymmetrical buttock that is mildly tender. The management of a suspected seroma is serial aspiration which may require several weeks to resolve. It is likely that most seromas are small enough that they are undetectable and resolve on their own. Large persistent seromas over 100 cc can present a problem if not addressed. Untreated seromas can become infected or lead to complications of implant malposition or extrusion as fluid dissects through tissue planes. Ultrasound can aid in the diagnosis of seroma. Seromas that fail to improve with serial aspiration should be cultured to evaluate for infection. Open drainage with washout and drain insertion may be indicated in these cases.

Capsular contracture is an uncommon complication of buttock augmentation with implants. The buttock may present as firm with an implant that is immobile. The shape of the buttock may not change as the semi-solid implant may resist the deformational pressure exerted by the capsule. The patient may complain of constant tightness and discomfort of the buttocks. Open exploration with capsulotomy may be indicated. Implant removal in severe cases may result in changes in buttock shape as the periprosthetic space collapses.

Aesthetic complications of buttock implant surgery may result from poor implant choice, surgical technique, or postoperative management. A poor aesthetic result due to implant selection could result from inserting a large oval implant into a short buttock resulting in rotation and asymmetry or from inserting a small round implant into a long buttock producing an empty inferior pole. Aggressive surgical dissection of the lateral or inferior aspect of the buttock can lead to palpability and visibility of the implant especially in the subfascial space. Under dissection of the inferior aspect of the buttock in the subfascial or intramuscular space can create high riding implants with a lack of central buttock projection and a deficient inferior pole. Subfascial implant insertion in a thin patient may produce unacceptable results as the soft tissue may not be able to accommodate the weight of an implant over time. Untreated infections, seromas or hematomas may lead to implant migration and displacement with thickening of the capsule and asymmetry with a high likelihood for the need for implant removal.

Revisional buttock implant surgery for aesthetic concerns should be performed at least 6 months postoperatively when the periprosthetic space has formed a stable capsule. At this time the tissues have relaxed and the implant may be exchanged for a larger size that would not have been able to be inserted originally.[31] Implants may also be exchanged to an oval or round shape to create a more pleasing aesthetic result. Site change should be considered for subfascial implants that that exhibit excessive palpability or visibility. Conversion to the intramuscular plane with an additional layer of coverage may eliminate these concerns. Displaced intramuscular implants can be reinserted into a new intramuscular space or stabilized with internal capsule suturing.[32,33] Secondary buttock implant surgery to replace implants removed for infection can be successfully performed provided that the buttock is free of infection or biofilm which usually requires a 6-month wait. If buttock implant reinsertion is not desired or possible fat grafting to the empty buttock can restore volume and symmetry.

23.5 Case Examples

23.5.1 Case 1

A 20-year-old woman 5 feet 5 inches tall weighing 115 pounds requesting enlargement of the buttocks. Note the lack of projection of the mid buttocks. Preoperative view (▶Fig. 23.6a–e) and postoperative results (▶Fig. 23.6a–e).

23.5.2 Case 2

A 22-year-old woman 5 feet 4 inches tall weighing 110 pounds requesting buttock enlargement. Preoperative view (▶Fig. 23.7a–e) and postoperative results (▶Fig. 23.7a–e).

23.5.3 Case 3

A 25-year-old woman 5 feet 8 inches tall weighing 106 pounds requesting buttock enlargement. Preoperative view (▶Fig. 23.8a–e) and postoperative results (▶Fig. 23.8f–j).

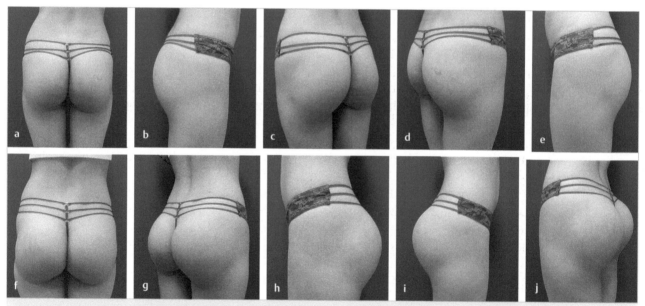

Fig. 23.6 (a–e) Preoperative views. Postoperative results **(f–j)** Seven months after subfascial insertion of round 276cc solid silicone implants via an intergluteal incision.
Note: Point of maximal projection at level of pubis in lateral views **(h, i)**.

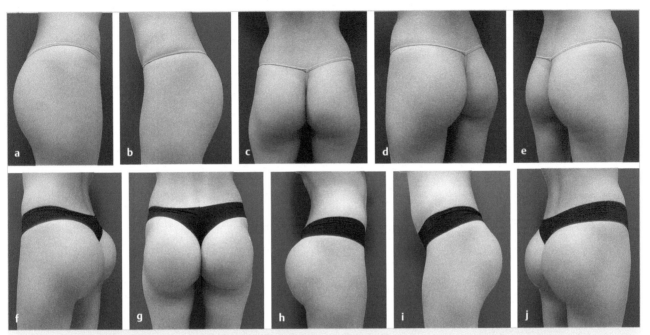

Fig. 23.7 Preoperative views **(a–e)**. 11 months after subfascial insertion of 276 cc solid silicone implants **(f–j)** postoperative results.
Note: Improvement in projection and global enhancement of the buttock.

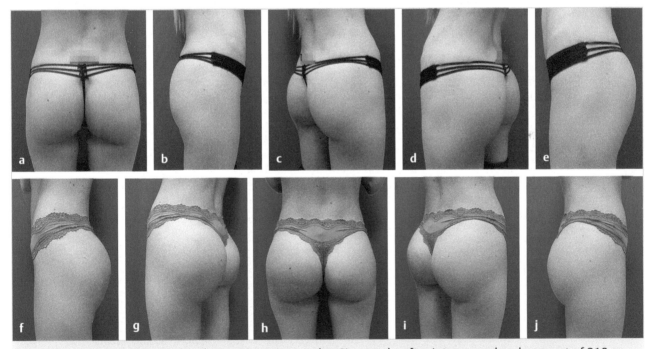

Fig. 23.8 Preoperative view **(a–e)**. Postoperative results: Six months after intramuscular placement of 218 cc round solid silicone implants **(f–j)**.
Note: Improvement in projection and volume of upper, central, and inferior aspect of the buttocks with slight widening of the lateral buttock region.

References

[1] Mendieta CG. Classification system for gluteal evaluation. Clin Plast Surg 2006; 33(3):333–346

[2] Centeno RF, Young VL. Clinical anatomy in aesthetic gluteal body contouring surgery. Clin Plast Surg 2006; 33(3):347–358

[3] Serra F, Aboudib JH, Cedrola JP, de Castro CC. Gluteoplasty: anatomic basis and technique. Aesthet Surg J 2010; 30(4):579–592

[4] Cuenca-Guerra R, Lugo-Beltran I. Beautiful buttocks: characteristics and surgical techniques. Clin Plast Surg 2006; 33(3):321–332

[5] Vergara R, Marcos M. Intramuscular gluteal implants. Aesthetic Plast Surg 1996; 20(3):259–262

[6] de la Pea JA. Subfascial technique for gluteal augmentation. Aesthet Surg J 2004; 24(3):265–273

[7] Bartels RJ, O'Malley JE, Douglas WM, Wilson RG. An unusual use of the Cronin breast prosthesis. Case report. Plast Reconstr Surg 1969; 44(5):500

[8] Cocke WM, Ricketson G. Gluteal augmentation. Plast Reconstr Surg 1973; 52(1):93

[9] Robles J, Tagliapietra J, Grandi M. Gluteoplastia de aumento: implante submuscular. Cir Plast Iberolatinoamericano 1984; 10:365–369

[10] de la Pea JA, Rubio OV, Cano JP, Cedillo MC, Garcs MT. History of gluteal augmentation. Clin Plast Surg 2006; 33(3):307–319

[11] Serra F, Aboudib JH, Neto JI, et al. Volumetric and functional evaluation of the gluteus maximus muscle after augmentation gluteoplasty using silicone implants. Plast Reconstr Surg 2015; 135(3):533e–541e

[12] Flores-Lima G, Eppley BL, Dimas JR, Navarro DE. Surgical pocket location for gluteal implants: a systematic review. Aesthetic Plast Surg 2013; 37(2):240–245

[13] Hwang SW, Nam YS, Hwang K, Han SH. Thickness and tension of the gluteal aponeurosis and the implications for subfascial gluteal augmentation. J Anat 2012; 221(1):69–72

[14] de la Pea JA, Rubio OV, Cano JP, Cedillo MC, Garcs MT. Subfascial gluteal augmentation. Clin Plast Surg 2006; 33(3):405–422

[15] Senderoff DM. Aesthetic surgery of the buttocks using implants: practice-based Recommendations. Aesthet Surg J 2016; 36(5):559–576

[16] Mofid MM, Gonzalez R, de la Pea JA, Mendieta CG, Senderoff DM, Jorjani S. Buttock augmentation with silicone implants: a multicenter survey review of 2226 patients. Plast Reconstr Surg 2013; 131(4):897–901

[17] Mezzine H, Khairallah G, Abs R, Simon E. [Buttocks enhancement using silicone implants: a national practices assessement about 538 patients] Ann Chir Plast Esthet 2015; 60(2):110–116

[18] Mendieta CG. Intramuscular gluteal augmentation technique. Clin Plast Surg 2006; 33(3):423–434

[19] Gonzalez R. Gluteal implants: the "XYZ" intramuscular method. Aesthet Surg J 2010; 30(2):256–264

[20] Gonzalez R, Mauad F. Intraoperative ultrasonography to guide intramuscular buttock implants. Aesthet Surg J 2012; 32(1):125–126

[21] Crdenas-Camarena L, Paillet JC. Combined gluteoplasty: liposuction and gluteal implants. Plast Reconstr Surg 2007; 119(3):1067–1074

[22] Roberts TL, III, Weinfeld AB, Bruner TW, Nguyen K. "Universal" and ethnic ideals of beautiful buttocks are best obtained by autologous micro fat grafting and liposuction. Clin Plast Surg 2006; 33(3):371–394

[23] Aiache AE. Gluteal re-contouring with combination treatments: implants, liposuction, and fat transfer. Clin Plast Surg 2006; 33(3):395–403

[24] Singh D. Universal allure of the hourglass figure: an evolutionary theory of female physical attractiveness. Clin Plast Surg 2006; 33(3):359–370

[25] Cardenas-Camarena L, Silva-Gavarrete JF, Arenas-Quintana R. Gluteal contour improvement: different surgical alternatives. Aesthetic Plast Surg 2011; 35(6):1117–1125

[26] Aboudib JH, Serra F, de Castro CC. Gluteal augmentation: technique, indications, and implant selection. Plast Reconstr Surg 2012; 130(4):933–935

[27] Bruner TW, Roberts TL, III, Nguyen K. Complications of buttocks augmentation: diagnosis, management, and prevention. Clin Plast Surg.2006; 33(3):449–466

[28] Senderoff DM. Buttock augmentation with solid silicone implants. Aesthet Surg J 2011; 31(3):320–327

[29] Mendieta CG. Gluteoplasty. Aesthet Surg J 2003; 23(6):441–455

[30] Vergara R, Amezcua H. Intramuscular gluteal implants: 15 years' experience. Aesthet Surg J 2003; 23(2):86–91

[31] Senderoff DM. Revision buttock implantation: indications, procedures, and recommendations. Plast Reconstr Surg In press

[32] Serra F, Aboudib JH. Gluteal implant displacement: diagnosis and treatment. Plast Reconstr Surg 2014; 134(4):647–654

[33] Jaimovich CA, Almeida MW, Aguiar LF, da Silva ML, Pitanguy I. Internal suture technique for improving projection and stability in secondary gluteoplasty. Aesthet Surg J 2010; 30(3):411–413

24 Technology-Based Contouring of the Thighs

W. Jason Martin

Abstract

Contouring procedures and treatments of the thighs that rely on invasive and noninvasive technologies, present a unique challenge to any level of surgeon. Technical competence notwithstanding, outcomes are often negatively influenced by the complex 3-dimensional anatomy of this region, the notable variance of patient clinical presentations and the inherent risk profile of the contouring technologies themselves. But mastery is not elusive. It is dependent on many pre-treatment and preoperative factors including the adequacy of the physical exam, the competent analysis of the patient's imaging, the reasonable management of a patient's expectations, and most importantly, the strength of the treatment plan that takes into account how well each technology works in the specific aesthetic subunits. Successful and reproducible outcomes should also be expected. Good results are largely dependent on the adequacy of the pretreatment and preoperative markings, the maintenance of patient comfort during the treatment or surgery, safe use of the contouring technology that systematizes patient positioning and a conservative approach to lipoplasty when included, especially when combined with technology based lipolysis. Lastly, post-treatment and postoperative care can be easily standardized and it should take into account the length of time for full results to be realized, up to 6+ months when laser-assisted lipolysis (LAL) or radiofrequency-assisted lipolysis (RFAL) is used.

Keywords: Laser-assisted lipolysis, radiofrequency-assisted lipolysis, VASER

24.1 Introduction

When considering the nascency of liposuction in the field of aesthetic surgery in the 1980s, Illouz's understanding of the complexities of lower extremity contouring procedures was remarkable. His delineation of the zones of adherence of the lower extremity (▶Fig. 24.1) and his descriptions of the associated blunt liposuction related complications (e.g., edema, ulceration, and hyperpigmentation) in these areas created a road map that plastic surgeons use to this day.[1] However, from the time of Illouz to present day, lower extremity contouring treatments and procedures have presented a special challenge to surgeons with a disproportionate number of average to unsatisfactory outcomes. Invariably multifactorial, this inherent difficulty does not often correlate to the surgeon's technical competency. Asymmetric localized adiposity, variable elasticity, contour deformities including cellulite, post-surgical deformities, skin abnormalities like striae and varicosities, heterogeneity of thigh fat and bilateral three-dimensional variances, are just a few of many factors that muddy the waters of a patient's clinical presentation. Add in the exploding field of invasive and noninvasive energy-assisted body contouring devices and the approach to thigh contouring has become more elaborate and progressively more confusing. Therefore, to truly master technology-based contouring of the thighs, one must be as facile and competent with the creation of a treatment plan as they are with the contouring treatments and procedures themselves.

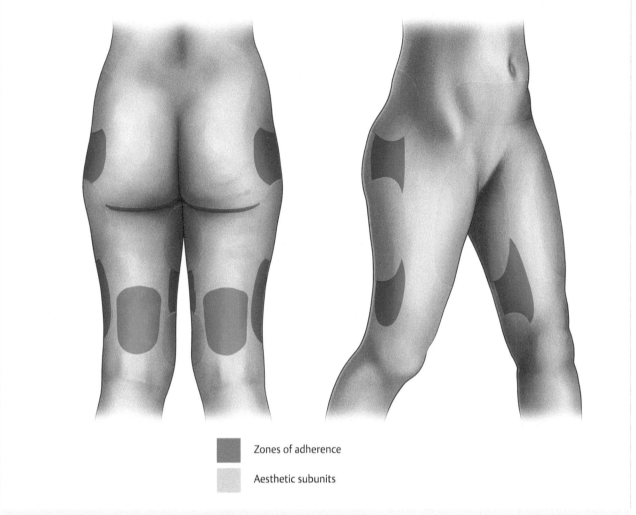

Zones of adherence

Aesthetic subunits

Fig. 24.1 Zones of adherence as described by Illouz.

As all aesthetic subunits of the lower extremities should be addressed en bloc, limiting your focus to one area will diminish the power of any treatment or procedure outcome. In the interest of clarity, this chapter will focus solely on the thighs, or the area of the lower extremities superior to the patella and popliteal fossa and inferior to the inguinal and gluteal crease.

24.2 Patient Evaluation

Evaluation of the thighs should always take into account the variable three-dimensional distribution of the superficial fat. As with the nose, assessing a complex three-dimensional anatomic location like the thigh for aesthetic purposes should incorporate aesthetic subunits. This author has found benefit in defining these subunits solely on the common areas of localized adiposity. This includes the medial thigh, lateral thigh, banana roll, upper 2/3rd of the anterior thigh, lower 1/3rd of the anterior thigh and the posterior thigh (▶ Fig. 24.2). The lateral portion of each thigh, inferior to the saddlebags, rarely has issues related to localized adiposity in a normal weight patient. The fat in this area is often fibrous and diminished along tensor fascia lata. In a similar fashion, the medial portion of each thigh, inferior to the medial thigh fat pad, usually has a paucity of superficial fat and should be approached with

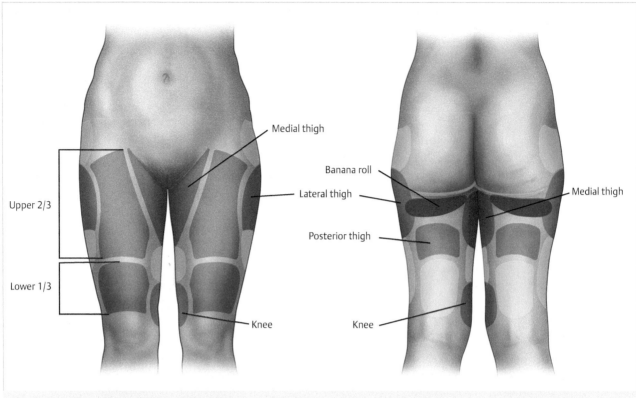

Fig. 24.2 Aesthetic subunits of the thigh.

care. It is important to note that the presentation of cellulite is often an outlier and is many times found in these medial and lateral zones. Therefore, when assessing cellulite alone, this author divides the thigh into four equal quadrants and then further divides each quadrant with a grid pattern.

The clinical exam should proceed as follows:

- A thorough review of the patient's pertinent past medical history including but not limited to surgical history, comorbid conditions, psychiatric history and current medications.
- A discussion of expectations related to a patient's thigh contour, both with and without clothes is essential to establishing realistic expectations. This should be completed before the exam so as to not to introduce bias.
- The physical exam should be completed both in a standing and sitting position. Furthermore, tangential lighting should be incorporated into the exam to better elucidate superficial contour deformities like cellulite.
- Photographic and/or three-dimensional imaging documentation during the initial clinical exam is highly recommended. Reviewing these images during the initial consult allows for a more constructive discussion with the patient regarding the treatment plan. In the author's practice, the images are projected to 1/2 life size proportions on the wall of the consulting room with overlay of diagramming, so that the patient can clearly visualize the areas of concern.

24.3 Preoperative Planning and Preparation

The treatment options for technology-based contouring of the thighs are plentiful. At the time of this publication, there were at least 15 noninvasive body-contouring devices that have FDA clearance or off label application for thigh contouring and at least Level 4 evidence from clinical studies using the American Society of Plastic Surgeons Levels of Evidence Rating Scale.[2] This does not include the multitude of devices and treatments, like injection lipolysis, that are just making their way to market for thigh contouring. A thorough review of noninvasive body-contouring devices can be found in Section 2 of this book. As integrating all of the devices into a clinic setting would not be feasible for even the largest practice, it is important to focus your practice's capital expenditure on diversity of treatment technology and the combination treatment potential. But make no mistake, the field of body contouring is heading in a less invasive direction and it is imperative to have at least one noninvasive device in your office. In the author's experience, treatment of superficial thigh localized adiposity with noninvasive body-contouring devices offers, at best, a 30% reduction in the treated fat. This is far removed from the efficacy of lipoplasty and should therefore not be presented as an equal alternative. Consider these devices adjunctive and a formative tool to potentiate lipoplasty results. Furthermore, as standalone treatments, they offer a powerful option for patients who are not good candidates for lipoplasty or those who do not desire a more invasive option. These options will vary per physician depending on their device lineup and their practice focus. Treatment settings should be adjusted per the clinical judgment of the physician and the recommendations from the manufacturer.

Technology based lipoplasty devices offer the most absolute treatment of localized adiposity of the thigh. A thorough description of these technologies can be found in this book. When developing a treatment plan for thigh contouring, it is useful to sort the application of these technologies by their usefulness in each aesthetic subunit and most importantly, by the skin quality in the treatment area. In general, ultrasound-assisted liposuction (UAL) and water-assisted liposuction (WAL) are more useful in large areas of debulking that have less skin elasticity concerns, like the upper 2/3rd of the anterior thigh and the majority of the posterior thigh. These technologies also have the added benefit of preserving the viability of adipocytes for autologous fat transfer, preserving the superficial lymphatic network thus decreasing postoperative edema and having the most desirable safety profile.[3,4] LAL and RFAL are more useful in areas of localized adiposity with variable levels of skin elasticity, like the medial thighs and lower 1/3rd of the anterior thigh. Although UAL technology like VASER does appear to have improved skin retraction in comparison to suction-assisted liposuction (SAL) (17% versus 10%), LAL devices like Smart Lipo and RFAL devices like Bodytite offer more potential for skin retraction (18 to 22% and up to 35% respectively).[3,5,6] Smart Lipo devices have the added bonus that Cellulaze can be added to the platform. Cellulaze is currently the most effective energy assisted invasive treatment option for cellulite.[7] Recommended application of each technology as it pertains to aesthetic subunits can be found in ▶ Fig. 24.3. Lastly, as each of these devices allows for improved treatment and recovery when compared to SAL, the primary focus should be on inclusion in a liposuction case, not exclusion based on an aesthetic subunit.

As with any aesthetic procedure, there should be a binal approach to preoperative planning, balancing patient expectations with the clinical presentation. Al la carte approach is discouraged as residual localized adiposity in untreated aesthetic subunits will diminish results. For areas that need less than 30% improvement, the patient is given the option between invasive or noninvasive modalities. For more notable levels of localized adiposity, technology based

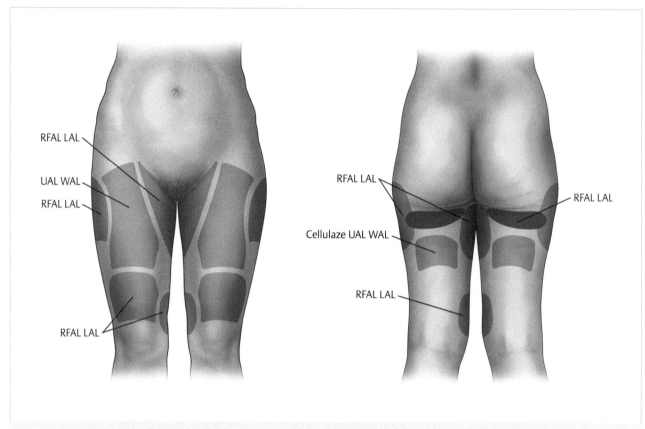

Fig. 24.3 Author's recommended technology in each aesthetic subunit.

lipoplasty is the treatment of choice. Progressive practices incorporate combination treatments of both invasive and noninvasive modalities. Furthermore, the noninvasive modalities are usually a patient's first introduction to the practice allowing for more meaningful marketing of the invasive options.

Exclusion criteria for liposuction and the requirements for office-based surgery is reviewed in Section 1. Thigh lipoplasty cases can be completed in the office setting unless combined with other procedures that require a higher degree of anesthesia. Diagramming on the preoperative photos is an important tool to finalize the surgical plan and is additive to the medical records.

24.4 Surgical Technique

A large majority of technology-based lipoplasty procedures of the thigh can be completed in the office setting with tumescent anesthesia. The author prefers to include additional oral analgesia and sedative-hypnotic agents for most of these cases. This includes Percocet (5–10/325) and Halcion 0.25 mg administered 30 minutes prior to surgical start time and after the surgical consent has been obtained. One of the benefits of awake procedures is that the anesthesia can be adjusted with input from the patient. Titration of these medications continues intraoperatively and second doses can be administered on a pro re nata basis. In combination cases that require an operative suite setting, intravenous sedation is the anesthesia of choice with a propofol infusion titrated to a desired level of sedation. In conjunction, versed is added preoperatively for anxiolysis, fentanyl is included for improved analgesia, and ketamine is often added for its dissociative properties. These agents are all titrated to achieve easy arousal at completion of the procedure and subsequent earlier discharge. If thigh liposuction is being combined with trunk contouring procedures like an abdominoplasty, regional anesthesia is a useful complement. Epidural catheters will lessen the demands for higher dose sedation and also decrease postoperative pain control requirements. The author's preference is that the patient is provided with an epidural in the lumbar region to cover associated dermatomes of the thigh. An alternative would be a single injection spinal anesthetic with an agent that has a shorter half-life. The local anesthetic doses administered by the anesthesiologist should be considered when calculating the total dose of local anesthetic administered during the case. To avoid toxicity in this setting, the lidocaine dosage in each bag of tumescent fluid is reduced by 50%. The epinephrine dose remains unchanged.

Surgical markings, in essence, are a projection of a surgeon's preoperative vision onto an animate form. When working through the complicated topography of the thigh, the process of surgical markings gives the surgeon a tactile and visual feedback that is essential for refinement of the approach. All markings are completed in a standing position and re-evaluated in a sitting position if necessary. Three-panel mirrors are also useful as they allow the patient to confirm the location of the markings with the surgeon. See ▶ Fig. 24.4 for examples of surgical markings in the different aesthetic subunits of the thigh. Dr. Pitman described a useful approach to lipoplasty markings where an area of localized adiposity is initially marked around its boundary and then divided into four equal quadrants.[8] This division allows the surgeon to monitor and ensure symmetrical aspiration from each quadrant thus reducing the risk of postoperative deformities. Depending on the location of the stab incision utilized in lipoplasty, the center point of the marked localized area of adiposity inherently has the highest risk for over aspiration due to the most number of cannula passes in this area. Encircling the confluence of the four quadrants gives the surgeon a useful visual reminder to avoid over aspiration in this area, thus decreasing the likelihood of postoperative surgical deformities.

Perioperative antibiotics are necessary and weight based dosing should be employed. This can be delivered orally or intravenously, depending on the anesthesia approach to the case. There is no persuasive clinical data supporting the usefulness of postoperative course of antibiotics. With this understood, the author still utilizes a seven-day oral course of postoperative antibiotics.

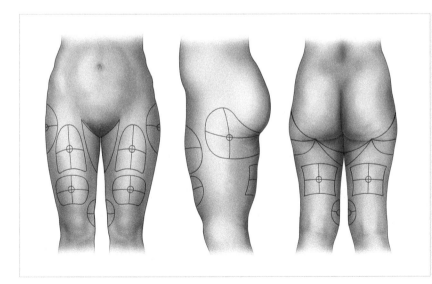

Fig. 24.4 Examples of surgical markings in each aesthetic subunits of the thigh.

Although the approach to a surgical prep can vary depending on the anatomic location, the author always utilizes a standing prep for lower extremity lipoplasty. This allows for easy access to all areas of the lower extremity and the patient is able to rotate each leg to further facilitate the prep. With a standing prep, sequential compression devices and intravenous catheters are placed on the upper extremity. Also, for patient comfort, the surgical prep should be maintained at or above room temperature with adherence to manufacturer recommendations. Before prepping, the surgical table is draped with a sterile sheet. After prepping, the patient is assisted onto the table with care taken to avoid contamination of the sterile sheet previously placed. Each lower extremity, below the knee, is carefully wrapped with a sterile sheet or covered with a sterile stockinette. Once this is completed and the rest of the body is sterilely draped, the patient's body can then be rotated and the lower extremities can be manipulated without compromising sterility. This freedom of maneuvering is critical to achieving successful results in lipoplasty of the thigh. One important point, with a standing prep, oral and intravenous anesthesia administration must be limited before prep initiation. It is imperative to inform the anesthesia and/or nursing staff in a timely fashion that a standing prep will be used. This avoids the safety concerns related to placing a patient in a standing position after administration of sedatives and anxiolytics.

Patient positioning preferences for lower extremity lipoplasty vary immensely depending on a surgeon's training. The author prefers to address the lateral thighs and the medial knees in a lateral decubitus position, the posterior thighs from a prone position, the medial thighs from a prone and supine frog-leg position, and the anterior thighs from a supine position. The stab incisions used for introduction of the lipoplasty cannula should be placed in anatomic creases like the gluteal fold or the inguinal crease when possible. Otherwise, due to the small size of the incision, placement of these incisions should improve a surgeon's ability to aspirate and deemphasize a location that is not visible with clothing. An #11 blade applied while the skin and soft tissue are pinched will result in an appropriately sized incision. Also, applying antibiotic ointment to the incision site will decrease the maceration injuries that occur from repeated skin contact with the lipoplasty cannula.

Injection of tumescent anesthesia with an awake patient in the office setting should be completed slowly from a deep to superficial plane (200 to 250 cc/minute). The author uses a flexible 18 gauge 6 hole infiltration cannula that is 27 cm in length. This smaller diameter cannula has much less discomfort when compared to the larger 14 gauge cannulas. Chapter 1 gives an in depth review of office based tumescent anesthesia and the recommended concentrations of the wetting solution. In general, the author prefers a Superwet technique (1:1 ratio for infiltrate and aspirate) with a max lidocaine dosage of 40 mg/kg. For each 1000 cc bag of 0.9% sodium chloride the assistant adds 100 cc of 1% lidocaine, 12 cc of 8.4% bicarbonate and 1 cc of epinephrine 1/1000. The total lidocaine dosage in each of these bags is 1000 mg which makes for more efficient visualization and recording of the injected dosage of lidocaine during the case. This is extremely important as lidocaine toxicity is an avoidable complication. In the operative setting that includes intravenous, inhalational, or regional anesthesia, the lidocaine dosage in each bag is reduced by 50%. This allows the surgeon to address more areas of localized adiposity without increasing the risk of lidocaine toxicity.

Technology-assisted treatment of the thighs should be completed before the initiation of lipoplasty. This is essential when using laser and RF assisted technology. Both of these technologies depend on the tumescent fluid acting as a heat sink, thus decreasing the incidence of dermal burns. In general, these technologies allow for more effective lipoplasty and therefore reinforce the importance of treating the areas of localized adiposity before aspiration. As the areas of localized adiposity of the thighs often concomitantly present with skin laxity, choosing technologies that further impart skin tightening in this area should be emphasized.

The recommended technique for aspiration follows a similar pattern in almost all areas of the thighs. Once the tumescent fluid has been injected, obtain a baseline by pinching the tissues encircled within the area of localized adiposity. Next insert the lipoplasty cannula and aspirate of the planned suction volume. Pinch the tissues again to evaluate the progress and highlight any irregularities by slowly running a hand over the surface. Carefully complete aspiration with care taken to avoid aggressive aspiration near the skin.[8] The selection of the aspiration cannula and the recommended plane of aspiration vary by each location. In areas of bulky localized adiposity like the saddlebags, lipoplasty is initiated in the deeper plane (greater than 1 cm from the skin) with a 4.0 mm 3 port radial Mercedes cannula 20 to 30 cm in length. Next, the more superficial plane (within 1 cm of the skin) is conservatively addressed with a 3.0 mm 3 port radial Mercedes cannula, 20 to 30 cm in length. In areas of mild to moderate localized adiposity, as with the medial thighs and knees, lipoplasty is maintained in a more superficial plane with a conservative amount of aspiration using a 2.5 to 3.0 mm 3 port radial Mercedes cannula 20 to 30 cm in length. For the anterior and posterior thighs, where the fat is not localized, a 3.0 to 4.0 mm 3 port radial Mercedes cannula 20 to 30 cm in length is recommended. A conservative approach is always necessary in these areas. Although the cannula tip should be maintained in a deeper plane to limit postoperative deformities, the surgeon must also be aware of the cannula tip location, avoiding important anatomic areas of concern like the popliteal fossa and femoral triangle. Lastly, aspiration volumes will vary for each area of localized adiposity depending on a patient's presentation and the amount of tumescent fluid utilized. Per the authors, experience, when using a superwet technique on an average patient (BMI < 30), the aspirate volumes often fall within a set range: saddlebags 300500 cc, medial thighs 100300 cc, medial knees 50100 cc and the anterior or posterior thighs 100200 cc. It is important to note that these aspiration volumes will vary depending on the technology employed with the lipoplasty procedure.

The importance of using preoperative markings as an intraoperative guide cannot be over emphasized. These markings allow the surgeon to use both visual cues and quantifiable data during the procedure. Specifically, using these markings as a guide, an assistant can maintain an intraoperative log that quantifies the aspirate volume for each area of localized adiposity, including the four marked quadrants. Having these measurements counters one of the primary causes of poor liposuction technique: an inability of the surgeon to visualize an area of asymmetry intraoperatively. And even as a surgeon's ability to grasp visual cues during lipoplasty improves with experience, the importance of quantifying aspirate amounts from each treatment area will remain unchanged. This becomes very evident when addressing localized adiposity of the lateral thighs in a lateral decubitus position. During these procedures, the recorded aspirate amount acts as a useful guide when switching from one side to the other as synchronous visualization is not feasible.

24.5 Results and Outcomes

24.5.1 Problems and Complications

Chapter 1 gives a comprehensive review of the risks associated with office based lipoplasty under local anesthesia. As it pertains to noninvasive body contouring and technology based lipoplasty devices, part two and part three of this book address the general risks and complications associated with each technology. It is the author's opinion that body contouring procedures of the thigh, especially when combined with technology assisted treatments or procedures, should be approached with caution. This is especially true with lipoplasty of the thigh, which has a higher incidence of postoperative complications when compared to most other anatomic areas.

The thigh offers a complex challenge when using devices that depend on thermal energy, like LAL and RFAL devices. Due to the complicated topography and a proclivity for thinner skin, there is an increased risk of thermal injuries in this area. This is especially true when you consider that the 3D contour of the thigh also encourages end hits of the device cannula with the deep dermis of the skin. End hits can have a disastrous effect on the skin due to the mechanical and thermal nature of the injury. It should be emphasized that thermal injuries are an avoidable complication, especially in the case of end hits, as it is almost always technique-driven. Therefore, when using these devices, ensure that the patient is properly positioned and confirm that all quadrants of the surgical field can be visualized. Utilize the non-dominant hand as a tactile guide near the tip of the cannula, providing reinforcement of the cannula depth. Incorporate continuous temperature monitoring when available and adhere to the treatment guidelines for the anatomic location as recommended by the manufacturer. If a thermal injury does occur conservative treatment is recommended and rarely is a surgical revision required.

Post lipoplasty contour deformities of the thigh can often be attributed to the inherent difficulty in assessing the thigh's 3D contour variances preoperatively and intraoperatively. Photographic analysis, including 3D imaging is helpful, but it does not guarantee surgical proficiency. The intraoperative evaluation is also limited as the tumescent fluid will distort the surgical field and mask asymmetries. These and other factors test a surgeon's technical abilities and surgical decision making. Therefore, rely on a well thought out surgical plan and embrace a more systematic approach to patient positioning. Ensure that the surgical markings are accurate and deliberate. Always be conscious of the cannula location in reference to the skin and the deeper structures. Most importantly, defer to a more conservative approach during aspiration, emphasizing bulk removal in the deeper tissue planes while sparing the more superficial layers.

References

[1] Illouz YG. Refinements in the lipoplasty technique. Clin Plast Surg 1989;16(2):217–233

[2] Nassab R. The evidence behind noninvasive body contouring devices. Aesthet Surg J 2015;35(3):279–293

[3] Nagy MW, Vanek PF, Jr. A multicenter, prospective, randomized, single-blind, controlled clinical trial comparing VASER-assisted Lipoplasty and suction-assisted Lipoplasty. Plast Reconstr Surg 2012;129(4):681e–689e

[4] Man D, Meyer H. Water jet-assisted lipoplasty. Aesthet Surg J 2007;27(3):342–346

[5] DiBernardo BE. Randomized, blinded split abdomen study evaluating skin shrinkage and skin tightening in laser-assisted liposuction versus liposuction control. Aesthet Surg J 2010;30(4):593–602

[6] Irvine Duncan D. Nonexcisional tissue tightening: creating skin surface area reduction during abdominal liposuction by adding radiofrequency heating. Aesthet Surg J 2013;33(8):1154–1166

[7] DiBernardo BE, Sasaki GH, Katz BE, Hunstad JP, Petti C, Burns AJ. A multicenter study for cellulite treatment using a 1440-nm Nd:YAG wavelength laser with side-firing fiber. Aesthet Surg J 2016;36(3):335–343

[8] Pitman GH. Thighs and buttocks. In: Pitman GH, ed. Liposuction and aesthetic surgery. St Louis: Quality Medical Publishing; 1993:337–385

25 Calf, Ankle, and Knee Contouring

Christopher T. Chia, Stelios C. Wilson, and Gerald H. Pitman

Abstract

The calf, ankle, and knee play an important role in the overall aesthetic appearance of the lower extremity. Further, these areas are often exposed while walking, standing, and sitting. These anatomic subunits require special consideration prior to contouring. Unlike more commonly treated areas, these areas have a relatively thin layer of fat which may lend itself to the potential for contour deformities. In this chapter, we offer our techniques for successfully, efficiently, and safely contouring these areas while minimizing contour deformities. Given the dependent nature of contouring below the knee, prolonged swelling can occur and thus a longer postoperative compression may be necessary when tolerated. When managed thoughtfully and with a knowledge of potential pitfalls, contouring of the calf, ankle, and knee can lead to pleasing results in properly selected patients.

Keywords: Body contouring, lower extremity contouring, liposuction, calf, ankle, knee

25.1 Introduction

Calves, ankles, and knees are anatomic areas of common concern to many patients who desire both cosmetic and functional benefits. Universally, strong thighs tapering to thinner calves and delicate ankles are considered to be desirable characteristics. In addition, thin knees without bulging are desired by all women as well. The appearance of excess knee adipose tissue, especially in the medial region, is exacerbated with the legs crossed. While they are amenable to suction-assisted lipectomy (SAL) to decrease bulk, craft a more sculpted leg profile, decrease edema and provide the ability to fit into certain styles of boots, calves, ankles, and knees remain a relatively uncommon area for treatment by most plastic surgeons. In properly selected patients, liposuction of these areas can be done reliably and reproducibly to provide high patient satisfaction.

25.2 Preoperative Evaluation

Full history and physical examination with a focus on the lower extremities with laboratory values and medical clearance obtained as needed is conducted as in any body contouring workup. More specifically, the surgical plan of the leg must be approached in a three-dimensional and circumferential manner which takes into consideration the differences in the relative amounts of skin, fat, muscle, and bone depending at what level the calf and ankle are operated. Patients will present with differing complaints as well as disparate areas of fat deposition. Due to the dependent position of the leg, postoperative swelling is prolonged compared to other areas of the body and may persist for six months or longer. Even with compression stockings, the patient should be made aware of this during consultation. During the physical examination and history, the surgeon seeks physiologic reasons for increased caliber of the leg which would be contraindications to liposuction. Lymphedema, incompetent veins, cardio-pulmonary causes of edema, and a host of other medical conditions must be first ruled out.

25.3 Markings

It is important to identify the muscular component contributing to the overall leg profile. In patients with particularly developed muscles especially with a low insertion of the soleus, the profile may not be significantly improved by fat removal. To differentiate this, the patient is examined in the "tip-toe" position so that the medial and lateral heads of the gastrocnemius muscle and soleus are easily identified and marked. If the distal Achilles tendon is short or the soleus muscle is wider than normal, for instance, a large improvement in contour with fat removal may not be possible. In contrast, removal of a relatively small volume of fat in patients with normal to long tendons can result in dramatic improvement in the profile. The distribution of fat also changes from more well defined proximally at the knee to more diffuse distally. It is noted that even in heavier patients, there is a paucity of fat overlying the anterior tibia and this is a region that rarely requires fat removal.

The head of the fibula is palpated and identified. Marking this clearly is important to determine the area which is not treated due to the proximity of a branch of the common peroneal nerve. Inadvertent contact by the instruments may causing neuropraxia and resultant foot drop and must be avoided. As mentioned above, the anterior pre-tibial area is marked with vertical lines as a region which rarely requires fat resection even in heavier patients. Any excess fat in the ankle region tends to be localized on either side of the Achilles tendon and overlying the medial muscle group. It is important to differentiate fat from muscle in this region using the simple pinch test.

Knees are treated medially where the excess bulging area marked in the standing position and exacerbated with outward rotation of the foot and the knee in flexion. This is generally medial to the patella and extends posteriorly to the border of the popliteal fossa. Superiorly, it extends to the quadriceps insertions and inferiorly to the medial tibial tubercle. For example, medial knee fat that is particularly visible with the legs crossed, is a good opportunity to improve a specific area of complaint while enhancing the overall leg profile in the standing position. The presence of the bony prominence of the femur exaggerates a relatively small amount of fat that, when resected, has a large impact. In contrast, the prepatellar fullness that is often accompanied with wrinkling should be approached with caution because the skin elasticity, presence of overlying quadriceps fullness, and excess fat may contribute to loss of support of the soft tissues if over-aggressive fat removal is undertaken.

25.4 Procedure

While commonly performed under general anesthesia, these areas readily lend themselves to the local anesthesia technique. In the latter situation, patients are given oral medications approximately one hour prior preoperatively to achieve adequate serum levels. They include an antibiotic, opioid pain medication, and benzodiazepine sedative. The tumescent solution of lidocaine and epinephrine are higher in concentration than with the patient asleep. In our practice, 1000 mg of lidocaine, 12 mL of sodium bicarbonate, and 1.5 mL of 1:1,000 concentration epinephrine is added to 1,000 mL of Ringer's lactate yielding a 0.10% concentration of lidocaine solution. Access incisions are injected with 1% lidocaine with 1:100,000 epinephrine and a 14 gauge needle is used to provide puncture access. In our experience, the circular puncture heals well with a minimal length while still being able to accommodate cannulas of varying sizes up to 5 mm diameter. In areas such as the knees, calves, and ankles, the smaller cannula sizes pair well with this technique. Tumescent infiltration may begin with a 20 gauge spinal needle for a 'first pass' analgesia application as the flow rate of tumescent correlates with the rate of soft tissue distension and hence pain. A blunt 16 or 18 gauze standard infiltration cannula is used to deliver the tumescent fluid first into the deep and intermediate subcutaneous fat space under low speed. The hydrostatic force is allowed to disperse the fluid throughout the adipose layer. Once the patient feels numb, the cannula is used to inject the more superficial fat layer and more nerve ending-rich subdermis until complete and dense analgesia is achieved.

Irrespective of the type of anesthesia, a standing, sterile preop 360 degrees of the entire lower extremity is required for accurate contouring so that all aspects of the leg are accessible. The feet are covered with sterile drapes or towels. If sequential compression devices are used for deep venous thrombosis prophylaxis, models that fit the feet underneath or applied to the upper extremities allow access to the leg.

Regarding positioning, the patient is placed prone so that the posterior aspect is approached first to access the majority of the fat over the gastrocnemius muscles as well as the medial and lateral aspects with the leg both extended and flexed. Under local anesthesia, the patient then can easily turn herself supine with the legs in the frog-legged position to access the medial/lateral aspects as needed while patients under traditional anesthesia are carefully turned in a coordinated and carefully orchestrated manner where the surgeon, anesthesiologist, and nursing staff turn the patient in one motion with maintenance of the airway as the priority. Limiting the incisions to the naturally occurring creases in the popliteal fossa for access to the knees and upper calves and low areas adjacent to the lateral and medial malleoli help to minimize visibility. Use of longer cannulas and instrumentation for both the tumescent and aspiration phases that extend from the knee to the ankles obviate the need for a midcalf access incision which would be much more readily seen.

When suctioning the knee with the leg extended, if too much fat is removed from the medial side resulting in a completely straight profile, a concavity will result when the patient is sitting with the leg flexed. Instead, place the patient in a slight frog-legged position with an access incision made in the posterolateral knee crease. The non-dominant hand is used to distract the soft tissues anteriorly to improve the angle with which the cannula is directed. The radial suctioning of the fat is at the level of the superficial fascia and aimed away from the popliteal fossa and its contents. The suprapatellar fat at the distal anterior end of the femur is a common area of complaint but care must also be taken to avoid over-resecting this area which may cause laxity of the overlying skin. It is worthwhile repeating that even though the excess fat is removed, the skin laxity over the patella may result in a wrinkled appearance.

Contouring of the calves and ankles requires a circumferential approach with localized fat resection relative to the musculoskeletal framework. The subcutaneous fat is relatively sparse and there is little margin for error especially at the distal end so even minor contour irregularities are easily seen. Smaller diameter cannulas are often used to effect gradual fat removal with less chance of over-resection. With the areas marked in unequal quadrants, access incisions proximally near the popliteal fossa and distally near the medial and lateral malleoli are used to infiltrate the soft tissues with tumescent with the patient in the lateral decubitus position. Here, the lateral fat compartments and the contralateral leg's medial fat compartments are treated. Upon completion of that side, the patient is carefully turned and the opposite areas are treated. In the awake patient, it is preferred to tumesce the entire leg because the patient easily moves herself with a 360 degree prep. Once the infiltration phases are complete, a combination of prone, decubitus, and supine positions are used to maximize the fat removal and contouring in a cylindrical approach. Checking and re-checking fat removal in multiple positions has a great advantage of ensuring even and symmetric contouring of the calves and ankles in the awake patient.

25.5 Postoperative Considerations

When compared to other areas, lower extremity liposuction involves a more prolonged postoperative swelling phase and the patients should be made aware. Stockings of medium compression (30 mm Hg) are worn for several weeks to months. 5–0 nylon sutures for closure of the access incisions are removed at ten days and leg elevation is required for at least the first 30 days following surgery. Heavy exercise and running are not allowed for 30 days postoperatively.

25.6 Pearls and Pitfalls

Pearls

- Circumferential sterile prep in the standing position ensures that a 360 degree access is available for accurate contouring of the entire leg.
- Make note of the knee and leg contour with the patient in the sitting position preoperatively to avoid over-resection.
- Local anesthesia option greatly simplifies the patient management intraoperatively with safe, quick positioning and easy access to multiple angles of approach to the different areas of the leg.
- Longer duration of compression leggings recommended due to the prolonged postoperative edema time of the dependent areas of treatment.

Pitfalls

- Marking of the fibular head preoperatively is important to identify the region where the branch of the peroneal nerve crosses superficially to avoid inadvertent nerve injury.
- The relatively thin fat layer lends itself to a slightly increased risk of contour deformities when compared to other anatomical areas and smaller diameter cannulas are recommended.
- Avoid aggressive removal of knee fat with the leg extended to avoid a concavity of the medial fat with the leg flexed in the sitting position.

Suggested Readings

Pitman GH. Liposuction and aesthetic surgery. Quality Medical Publishing, Inc.; 1993:413445

Watanabe K. Circumferential liposuction of calves and ankles. Aesthetic Plast Surg 1990; 14(4):259–269

Reed LS. Lipoplasty of the calves and ankles. Clin Plast Surg 1989;16(2):365–368

Mladick RA. Lipoplasty of the calves and ankles. Plast Reconstr Surg 1990; 86(1):84–93, discussion 9496

Ilouz Y-G. Body contouring by lipolysis: A 5-year experience with over 3,000 cases. Plast Reconstr Surg 1984;73:780–794

Index

Note: Page numbers set in **bold** or *italic* indicate headings or figures, respectively.